I0222637

OMAD DIET

Omad- Friendly Recipes for a Balanced and Healthy Diet

(Easy Recipes to Attain Weight Loss)

Ellen McClinton

Published by Alex Howard

© **Ellen McClinton**

All Rights Reserved

Omad Diet: Omad- Friendly Recipes for a Balanced and Healthy Diet (Easy Recipes to Attain Weight Loss)

ISBN 978-1-77485-010-7

All rights reserved. No part of this guide may be reproduced in any form without permission in writing from the publisher except in the case of brief quotations embodied in critical articles or reviews.

Legal & Disclaimer

The information contained in this book is not designed to replace or take the place of any form of medicine or professional medical advice. The information in this book has been provided for educational and entertainment purposes only.

The information contained in this book has been compiled from sources deemed reliable, and it is accurate to the best of the Author's knowledge; however, the Author cannot guarantee its accuracy and validity and cannot be held liable for any errors or omissions. Changes are periodically made to this book. You must consult your doctor or get professional medical advice before using any of the suggested remedies, techniques, or information in this book.

Table of contents

Part 1

Introduction

The World Health Organization (WHO) defines obesity as abnormal or excessive fat accumulation that presents a risk to health. Obesity is a health concern, as it is a risk factor for many common chronic diseases such as heart disease and stroke, diabetes mellitus, osteoarthritis, and hypertension. The WHO estimates that being overweight or obese leads directly to the death of at least 2.8 million adults every year worldwide. Current guidelines use the body mass index (BMI) to define obesity. All adults aged 20 years and older are evaluated on the same BMI scale as Follows:

• Underweight: BMI below 18.5

• Normal weight: BMI 18.5 to 24.9

• Overweight: BMI 25.0 to 29.9

• Obese: BMI 30 and above

In addition to calculating your BMI, measuring body fat percentage is a good way to determine weight status. BMI factors in only your height and weight. It will give you the same reading if you have 160 N pounds of pure muscle or 160 pounds of pure fat. Body fat percentage is the percentage of weight that is pure fat.

The tendency toward a body type with an unusually high number of fat cells—termed endomorphic—

appears to be inherited. Other genetic factors influence appetite and the metabolic rate at which food is transformed into energy. Although inheritance may play a role, a genetic predisposition toward weight gain does not in itself cause obesity. Family eating habits are major contributors to the development of obesity.

Chapter 1: one meal a day; a neccesity?

Proper eating habits are the most important factor involved in losing weight permanently. We need to follow the eating habits of our ancestors, the hunter-gatherers, to maintain our health and body weight.

For our ancestors, it was feast or famine. Humans have evolved to endure long periods of time without food. Most cultures around the world eat one, two, or three times per day and do not snack between meals. People in wealthy, developed countries have access to food whenever they want. This has led people to become "grazers" and to eat whenever they feel like. Snacking is common and snack foods are readily available. In recent years, some nutritional experts have recommended grazing or having five or six "mini meals," making people believe that this is a healthy eating habit. However, there are no studies to support this way of eating, and there is actually plenty of evidence against it.

In the short term, eating small, frequent meals every day may help those with hypoglycemia by stabilizing their blood sugar. These people feel good for a while. However, eventually—usually between six and nine months—people notice that they feel hungry all the time. They gain weight and can't seem to lose it.

FREQUENCY OF MEALS

In an effort to combat the obesity epidemic, for many years scientists and medical experts have been trying to find the secret to weight loss. Finally, groundbreaking research has found the answer, and it's so simple that it may easily be overlooked. However, sometimes the simple solutions are the most powerful. Human nature, with its ego, tends to complicate everything, essentially making solutions to problems harder to find. As Albert Einstein said, "Everything should be made as simple as possible, but not simpler."

The secret to losing weight and keeping it off, as well as to improving one's health, is reducing eating freꝗuency. If you get only one thing out of this book, keep this in mind: Eat only once per day and do not have any snacks at all.Losing weight is as simple as eating only once daily, not consuming any snacks, and skipping dinner (or, if you are hungry, drinking a broth soup for dinner). Once you achieve your weight-loss goal you may decide to have a solid, light dinner eaten two or three hours before bedtime. In a study comparing two meals per day to six meals per day, researchers found that eating only breakfast and lunch reduced body weight, fastingvplasma glucose, C-peptide, and glucagon more than did eating the same amount of food spaced out over six meals. The group eating two meals a day ate their first meal between 6 a.m. and 10 a.m. and the next meal between 12 p.m. and 4 p.m.

The group eating six meals per day ate at regular intervals throughout the day. Despite consuming the same number of calories, the group eating only two meals a day lost, on average, three pounds more than the snackers did and about 1.5 inches more from around their waists. The participants eating six meals per day felt less satisfied and hungrier than did those eating only twice per day.

Most cultures around the world eat only two or three meals per day and do not eat snacks. The skinny French and Chinese cultures do not snack at all or do so very rarely. It is a widespread but scientifically unproven belief that eating small, fre uent meals is in some way beneficial. Recent research has found that spreading out food intake into smaller, more fre uent meals is associated with weight gain and does not have any beneficial effects on weight or health in the long term.In fact, research shows that eating more than three times a day is a factor that causes weight gain and obesity in the long term.

There is a growing body of scientific evidence to support the health and weight-loss benefits of reduced meal fre uency, meal timing, and intermittent fasting. Reduced meal frequency has been shown to suppress the development of various diseases.

The rhythm of eating only one or two times per day around the same time each day teaches the body to experience real hunger followed by fullness and satisfaction. Eating more than three times per day— whether it's a meal, a snack, a sugary drink, alcohol, caffeine, or anything else that raises blood sugar— leads to weight gain.

If you are used to eating frequently, slowly work your way down to less frequent eating. For example, start with four meals a day, then work your way down to three, and then two. Finally, if possible, try eating only once per day.

Make the extra effort to sit down, relax, and enjoy each meal. Focus on the food you are eating and on nothing else: no watching television, talking on the phone, standing when you eat, driving, or using a laptop. It may feel strange at first, but you will eat less, digest better, and enjoy your food more.

Once you have reached your ideal weight, you can maintain it effortlessly by eating no more than three times per day and by not snacking.

TIMING OF MEALS

Proper meal timing, as well as the amount of calories consumed at each meal, are more important than many people realize. A study found that the best mealtimes are breakfast around 7 a.m., lunch around 12:30 p.m., and a light dinner around 6 p.m. The study also found that breakfast is the most important meal of the day and that skipping breakfast leads to hunger and overindulgence later in the day.

Eating a large, satisfying breakfast every single day has helped dieters reduce their calorie intake throughout the day. Dinner should be the lightest meal of the day and should be eaten at least three hours before bedtime.

Dinner must be eaten early, not later than 7 p.m., because people are generally less active in the evening, causing extra calories to turn into fat. Researchers conducted a 20-week study to examine the effect of meal timing on weight loss. In one group, study participants consumed a breakfast that provided the day's highest amount of calories. In a second group, dinner provided the day's highest amount of calories. Researchers found that having the main meal of the day at breakfast time led to weight loss throughout the 20 weeks and that this effect was independent of total 24-hour calorie intake.

A follow-up study done for 12 weeks showed that those who had their main meal and higher calorie intake at breakfast time lost more weight than did those assigned to a higher calorie intake at dinner.

A study found that those who consumed an early lunch (before 3 p.m.) lost 4.85 pounds more than did those who ate lunch later.

Another study found that eating lunch at 4:30 p.m. decreased metabolism and glucose tolerance as compared to a lunch at 1 p.m.

 Eating an early lunch is the custom in many rural parts of France.

DRINK A SOUP FOR DINNER

Dinner should be the lightest meal of the day. When you are trying to lose weight, skip dinner altogether. If you are really hungry, drink a broth soup or have a liquid meal for dinner. Dinner must be eaten early because people are less active in the evening, and extra calories are more likely to turn into fat.

Most overweight people are unable to estimate proper portion sizes, which results in excessive calorie intake. Therefore, to limit excess food and calorie intake at dinnertime, drink a liquid meal. Studies have found that liquid meals help individuals lose weight.

Eating the majority of your calories at breakfast and the least amount of your calories at dinner in liquid form is an effective way to lose weight because fat storage is greatest in the evening.One of the main reasons the French stay so slim is that they eat very lightly at dinner. The French typically have a very light dinner, with little more than a bowl of soup and a salad. In countries ranking low in rates of obesity, such as Spain and Sweden, residents typically eat their biggest meals at lunchtime. For many Americans, dinner tends to be the biggest and most calorie-dense meal of the day.

Marie Antoinette, the 18th-century French Queen (1755-1793) ate cake for breakfast. Butter, milk, and cream were part of her daily diet. However, she stayed slim, with a waist size of 23 inches. She remained slim even after the birth of four children. Her first secret was that she ate only two meals per day. Her second secret was that she ate the majority of her calories during breakfast and lunch, and consumed soup for dinner, a French custom termed "souper." If eating a big breakfast doesn't suit your lifestyle, you can eat the majority of your calories at lunch. Marie Antoinette indulged her sweet tooth in the mornings, had her main meal consisting of meat or fish and vegetables at lunchtime and then had broth soup for dinner.

Many people wonder why they eat late at night and wake up feeling groggy and run down the next morning. The reason for this is that their circadian rhythms become disrupted when they eat late at night. In their early development, humans did not have access to food around the clock. They cycled through periods of feast and famine, and modern research shows that this cycling is the way we are meant to eat. By adjusting the timing of when you eat, you can dramatically alter your health and weight. If you are really hungry, you can consume a high-quality, organic, commercially prepared liquid meal for dinner, or drink a homemade soup made of nothing but vegetables and bone broth (no noodles, rice, or meat). However, you will sleep better and have more energy in the morning if you skip dinner altogether.

The soup that Marie Antoinette drank for dinner is prepared by boiling chicken, turkey, lamb, or beef bones for several hours. The long boiling time releases minerals from the bones. Vegetables such as onion, garlic, celery, kale, chard, and carrots are added, as well as turmeric and herbs, and each bowl contains around 100 calories. The soup can be prepared in advance and frozen in batches that can be quickly reheated when you are tired at the end of a busy day.

HEALTHY EATING HABITS

Properly timing meals and eating less frequently is important for everyone who wants to remain healthy and have energy, not only for people who want to lose weight.

According to the Centers for Disease Control and Prevention (CDC), nearly 90 percent of adults who have prediabetes don't know they have it. Prediabetes results from eating too frequently and eating high-sugar foods. In 2002, the New York Academy of Sciences published a report stating that all-day grazing can put a person at risk for type 2 diabetes, heart disease, and stroke. The risk increases when insulin spikes after consumption of foods that have high glycemic values. "If you eat only one to two meals a day, your insulin levels have time to even out," says Victor Zammit, head of cell biochemistry at Hannah Research Institute in Ayr, Scotland.

Freᵭuent eating puts pressure on the pancreas, never giving it a rest. When insulin levels are driven again and again many times a day, the pancreas becomes worn out and the cells can become resistant to taking in any more sugar.

The controlled timing of food intake and eating only one meal per day has been found to be the best way to eat if you have diabetes. In a study by Hanna Fernemark and colleagues comparing a low-fat diet, a low-carbohydrate diet, and a one-meal-per-day Mediterranean diet, it was found that if a person has type 2 diabetes, one massive meal per day is better than several smaller meals. The one-meal-per-day diet included one cup of black coffee for breakfast at 8 a.m. and a large Mediterranean-style lunch at 11:30 a.m. with a glass of wine.

Natural health, Ayurveda, and sports medicine expert Dr. John Douillard states that eating too frequently can result in blood sugar problems, weight gain, and a host of other problems.

He explains that when you eat six times a day, you create insulin spikes and, over time, lose the ability to burn fat effectively. This also leads to insulin resistance. When you eat every two or three hours, your body will burn fuel from those meals or snacks, but it will not burn any of its stored fat for energy. "If you have a healthy snack, like a carrot, in between breakfast and lunch you will burn the carrot but you will not burn any stored fat between those two meals," says Dr. Douillard.

Eating only one to three times per day is essential because, during the five or more hours between meals, the body is forced to burn stored fat. Whatever you eat turns into blood sugar, so every time you eat, your blood sugar goes up. To keep blood sugar stable, you must eat less frequently.

Insulin is the primary hormone that works to put on fat. By controlling your insulin and keeping it low, you can lose weight. "Eating breakfast, lunch and supper with no snacks in between will provide a natural fast in between meals that will encourage fat metabolism," says Dr. Douillard. After following this eating habit, you will notice "better energy, more stable moods, greater mental clarity, better sleep, fewer cravings and of course, natural and permanent weight management."

For his book The 3-Season Diet, Dr. Douillard conducted a study in which he instructed a group to eat three meals a day with no snacks, then measured weight loss and a host of psychological factors. Within two weeks, members of the group experienced better moods, fewer cravings, improved sleep, and less exhaustion after work. They also lost an average of 1.2 pounds per week throughout the two-month study.

INTERMITTENT FASTING

Intermittent fasting has become popular due to the growing research in its favor. Several books have been published on the topic. It typically consists of a very low-calorie allowance on alternate days (ADF) or two days a week (5:2 diet). Normal eating is resumed on non-diet days. It is a simple concept, which makes it easy to follow with no difficult calorie counting every other day. Intermittent fasting works to promote weight loss, but is linked to hunger during the fasting days (very low-calorie days).

Essentially, fasting means eating nothing and drinking only water for a certain period of time. Deliberate fasting is practiced worldwide, mostly for traditional, cultural, or religious reasons. It has been shown that fasting for the biblical period of 40 days and 40 nights is well within the overall physiological capabilities of a healthy adult. Some believe that intermittent fasting will shift your body into "starvation mode." Starvation mode is a scare tactic that the food and health industry uses to keep people fat. However, a study found that there was no change in the metabolic rates of people after 60 consecutive hours of fasting, and even after those 60 hours the reduction of the metabolic rate was only eight percent. Intermittent fasting increases insulin sensitivity. It has been found that intermittent fasting is more effective for weight loss than is traditional calorie restriction. Fasting is a powerful detoxification method, proven to remove toxins from the body. The scientific term for detoxification is autophagy. Autophagy means that your body flushes out everything it doesn't need. This happens at the cellular level. Cells consume their defective parts. Autophagy is essential for detoxifying cells and guaranteeing their proper function.If we eat all the time, our cells never get a chance to detoxify and rebuild themselves. Cells cannot break down defective parts and absorb materials to build new cell parts at the same time, so fasting for certain periods is essential to encourage the process. Research reveals that when animals and people are allowed to eat as they please, very little autophagy occurs. Even a tiny snack is enough to stop this process of cellular repair. In the absence of this important repair mechanism, defects in the cell can accumulate, causing disease and accelerated aging.

There is a large body of research to support the numerous health benefits of fasting. Fasting reduces the risk of type 2 diabetes, cardiovascular disease, cancer, and neurodegenerative disorder Fasting has also been proven to delay aging and increase lifespan. Many people carry out fasting in conjunction with intestinal cleansing through enemas or colonics to increase the healing effect that fasting provides.

There is significant empirical and observation-based evidence that medically supervised fasting spanning periods of 7 to 21 days is effective in the treatment of chronic diseases such as rheumatic diseases, chronic pain syndromes, hypertension, and metabolic syndrome.

Fasting also improves thinking ability, depression, insomnia, and anxiety. Gabriel Cousins, MD states, "I often observe in the fasting participants that by four days of [full-day] fasting, concentration seems to improve, creative thinking expands, depression lifts, insomnia stops, anxieties fade, the mind becomes more tranⓆuil and a natural joy begins to appear. It is my hypothesis that when the physical toxins are cleared from the brain cells, mind-brain function automatically and significantly improves and spiritual capacities expand."

Abstaining from food for even one full day (24 hours) is difficult for some people and not suitable for everyone. There are different types of fasts and different ways to abstain from food for a period of time. You can improve your health and lose weight without taking on full-day fasts. Fasting overnight might have similar benefits to full-day fasts.

By eating only once per day and eating as much as you want at that time,you can take part in fasting without going hungry. For example, by eating breakfast at 7 a.m. or eating lunch at 1 p.m. and by not eating dinner (except for a broth soup if you feel hungry), you are fasting from 1 p.m. until 7 a.m. the next day, which is 16 hours of fasting. If you don't eat for 12 to 16 hours, your body will go to its fat stores for energy. You will then break the fast with "break-fast."

CONTROL INSULIN TO BURN FAT

The cells of the body need sugar for energy. However, sugar cannot get into most cells directly. After a meal, a rise in blood sugar levels signals cells in the pancreas, called beta cells, to secrete insulin, which pours into the bloodstream. Insulin signals cells to absorb sugar from the bloodstream. Within 20 minutes after a meal, insulin rises to its peak level. If there is more sugar in the body than it needs, insulin helps store the sugar in your liver.

In healthy people, two to three hours after a meal, insulin levels return to a baseline and the pancreas makes a different hormone called glucagon. This hormone tells your liver to release the sugar it has stored to sustain your blood sugar levels. Just as insulin signals the fed state, glucagon signals the starved state.

It serves to mobilize glycogen stores from the liver when there is no food intake.

Gluconeogenesis typically begins four to six hours after the last meal and becomes fully active as stores of the liver's glycogen are depleted. It's during gluconeogenesis that your body will burn your stored fat for fuel.

If you eat a snack or another meal within six hours of eating, insulin rises again, which inhibits fat burning. You are supposed to get a snack between meals, but it should come from your fat stores, not from the consumption of food. Eating a large dinner or eating after dinner makes matters even worse because sleep is a prime opportunity to burn fat. When the body is fed every two to three hours, it uses fuel from those meals instead of burning its fat stores. The body adapts to being fed constantly without needing to dig into its fat stores. However, when you eat one or two meals a day and don't snack in between, the body is forced to burn its fat. "If you snack just as your insulin blood level is decreasing, it will promptly rise, even if you have a good snack such as fruit and nuts," says Eduardo Castro, MD, a specialist in fat-loss resistance syndrome. Eating frequently keeps insulin levels elevated constantly, which makes your body continually store fat.

High insulin levels inhibit the body's fat burning ability. You must keep insulin secretion low. Low levels of insulin allow your body to produce large amounts of lipase, the hormone responsible for releasing fat into your bloodstream to be used as fuel. You want to finish eating each meal within an hour or less and not eat your next meal until six or seven hours have passed. This means not eating or drinking anything that will prompt insulin release until your next meal.

Caffeine, tea, a sugary drink, or a small snack will prompt insulin release. If you drink coffee, tea, freshly squeezed fruit juice, or any beverage besides water, consume them during meals, not in between meals. Commercially prepared fruit juices such as apple juice or orange juice are the worst, as they are very high in sugar and quickly raise blood sugar levels. If you have problems with digestion (gas, bloating, burping, low energy after eating), drink bone broth or lacto-fermented beverages with your meals.

They assist in the digestion and assimilation of nutrients.

EAT LESS OFTEN

Eating only once per day and consuming absolutely no snacks will not only help you lose weight permanently, it will dramatically improve your health. A groundbreaking study compared the weight and health effects of two groups of people eating the same high-calorie diet. One group ate only three times per day, while the second group ate more frequently and consumed snacks. The group that ate frequently accumulated belly fat and developed nonalcoholic fatty liver disease, while those eating only three times per day did not. The study suggests that snacking contributes to weight gain and nonalcoholic fatty liver disease. This study surprisingly reveals that those eating a high-calorie diet in only three meals do not experience the negative effects on their health or weight that people eating more frequently do. Another study found that eating during specific times (time-restricted feeding) decreases body weight, lowers concentrations of triglycerides, glucose, and low-density lipoprotein (LDL) cholesterol, and increases concentrations of high-density lipoprotein cholesterol.

Scientists have discovered that reduced meal frequency can prevent the development of diseases and increase the lifespan of laboratory animals.

If you are unable to eat less frequently because of gnawing hunger and cravings for food, there are hidden health factors that you need to address.

A HIGH-FAT DIET

The U.S. Department of Agriculture (USDA) noted in 2013 that fat consumption has declined in the United

States in the last few decades, but rates of obesity have not gone down. Surprisingly, recent research has found that it's not so much what you eat, but when you eat it. Disruption of circadian rhythms by eating ad libitum (eating at any time of the day) is the problem that leads to obesity and metabolic disorders. The circadian clock regulates the expression and activity of certain metabolic enzymes, hormones, and transport systems.

Time-restricted feeding limits the time and duration of food availability (meal frequency). A study found that mice confined to specific time restricted periods of eating a high-fat diet became leaner and healthier than mice that ate the same diet but ate whenever they wanted. The mice on the time-restricted feeding schedule consumed an equivalent amount of calories from a high-fat diet as did those with unlimited access, yet were protected against obesity, hyperinsulinemia, fatty liver, and inflammation.

Mice fed a time-restricted, high-fat diet had much better satiation, 18 percent lower body weight, 30 percent decreased cholesterol levels, 10 percent reduced TNF-levels (tumor necrosis factor involved in systemic inflammation), and improved insulin sensitivity as compared to the group of mice fed a low-fat diet, ad libitum. This is very interesting because the amount of calories per gram of food was higher in the high-fat diet. The time restricted, high-fat diet group had no caloric restrictions, yet lost more weight than did the mice fed a low-fat diet, ad libitum.In another study of a structure similar to that of the previously mentioned study, time-restricted feeding caused less weight gain than did all-hour food access for mice eating a high-fat, high-sugar diet over 12 to 26 weeks. Interestingly, time-restricted feeding of a high-fat diet actually led to weight loss of up to 12 percent when applied to mice that were already obese.

Chapter 2: make it work

If you are used to eating fre∅uently and snacking, it is suggested that you gradually improve your eating habits. Start by eating only four meals a day, four hours apart, and work your way down to three meals. Eventually, work your way down to only one solid meal a day and if you are really hungry only drink a bone broth soup for dinner.

Children, teenagers, young adults, bodybuilders, and athletes, or those with an exceptionally fast metabolism, are able to eat more frequently without gaining weight. However, with age, their eating habits will likely catch up to them, and they can develop health issues related to bad eating habits such as snacking and eating frequently.

The following testimonial comes from the book, Secrets from the Eating Lab, and attests to eating only two meals per day. When he was younger, a man had raised a pig for the state fair. He fed his pig only twice per day, allowing the pig to eat as much as it wanted during its two meals. His friends fed their pigs the traditional way, letting the pigs have access to food all day long and allowing them to eat whenever they wanted. When it came time for judging, the man's pig had grown to be very lean, strong, and healthy, while his friends' pigs had grown fat.

Pigs are not known for their lean figures; therefore, the man who had raised the lean pig, who himself was overweight, was convinced that he had found the secret to losing weight and keeping it off. He decided to eat only twice per day. He ate as much as he wanted and ate whatever he wanted, but he ate only twice per day. He lost 42 pounds in two years and has kept it off for seven years and counting.

As easy as the eating less fre🞎uently sounds, each individual is unique and will have to find a way to make this strategy work for his or her situation and lifestyle. Time, work schedule, willpower, and other factors need to be considered. For some, it's very difficult to eat only once per day, and they need two or three meals. However, three meals should be the maximum amount of meals allowed.

DIET

The foundation of a healthy diet is consuming low GI and low-GL foods. Studies show that low GI and low GL diets promote weight loss. Although low-carbohydrate, high-protein diets have become popular means of losing weight, there is a large body of evidence that indicates low GI diets are the best way to lose weight and prevent diseases such as diabetes and cardiovascular disease.

A HEALTHY DIET

Most weight-loss diets are unbalanced and unhealthy, eliminating certain foods or food groups (carbs, protein, fats) that are essential to long-term good health. The only foods a person should eliminate from his or her diet are those they can't tolerate (e.g., cow's milk because of allergic reactions, or gluten because of celiac disease). Carbohydrates, fats, and protein are all important components of a balanced, healthy diet. A good rule of thumb is to divide your plate in the following way at each meal: one-half vegetables, one-quarter protein, and one-quarter whole grains or starches. In other words, 50 percent veggies, 25 percent protein, and 25 percent whole grain or another healthy starch.

According to extensive research into the healthiest cultures, the ideal diet consists of mainly organic produce, whole grains, pulses, seeds, nuts, fish, meat, and dairy. It also entails the avoidance of foods detrimental to one's health, including sugar, white flour, and foods not suitable for a person due to allergies or other individual factors.

It is important to consume a variety of whole foods and not eat the same foods day after day. It is important to vary your diet to make sure you are covering all your nutritional bases. It may be possible for some people to develop intolerances to foods eaten too often. For example, some people have developed food sensitivities to their favorite foods because they ate them on a daily basis for long periods of time.

Most studies show that reducing healthy fats is harmful. Some people think that they are doing their health good by replacing butter with margarine and by eliminating eggs and red meat from their diets. However, Dr. Weston Price found that the world's healthiest cultures ate protein in the form of organ meats and dairy products and considered animal fats absolutely essential to good health.

Their diets consisted of healthy fats, meats, fruits, vegetables, legumes, nuts, seeds, lacto-fermented foods, bone broth, and whole grains in their whole, unrefined state, as well as some raw foods of both animal and vegetable origin. This is what a healthy, balanced diet should be composed of. Dr. Price found that people eating this diet were free of disease, dental decay, and mental illness. When they started to consume an unhealthy, typical Western diet, their health rapidly deteriorated. He found that consumption of refined grains, canned foods, hydrogenated fats, refined oil, sugar, and pasteurized milk spoils our God-given inheritance of physical perfection and vibrant health.

HUNGRY FOR CHANGE

Everyone who wants to lose weight, feel better, have more energy, and get healthier should watch the documentary Hungry for Change (2012). The documentary discusses the real cause of weight gain and why diets don't work. It exposes shocking secrets the diet, weight loss, and food industries don't want you to know. Some of the key points are:

Diets do not work. Ninety to ninety-five percent of people who go on a diet will not only regain their weight but gain back even more.

Foods in modern societies are high in calories and low in nutrients. On the other hand, in healthier traditional cultures, whole foods are high in nutrients and generally low in calories.

Many people in America are chronically overfed but undernourished. Being chronically starved of nutrients causes a person to constantly eat in an effort to fulfill their body's requirements for nutrients.

People in modern societies are not eating real, whole foods, but rather food-like products such as boxed, packaged, canned foods, weight loss drinks, and food bars.

Many packaged foods are now touted as having zero calories, no fat, and no sugar. However, this is simply a marketing ploy. For example, foods marketed as low-fat can contain plenty of sugar, and sugar converts easily into fat. Foods marketed as having zero calories and no sugar typically have many toxic artificial sweeteners that cause weight gain in the long run.

Food companies are similar to tobacco companies. They know that if they addict a customer, they have that customer for life. Consequently, they use various chemicals that are known to cause addiction: monosodium glutamate (MSG), processed sugar, and artificial sweeteners. They put chemicals in their

food so that people keep buying it. Artificial sweeteners such as aspartame are very toxic and contribute to weight gain in the long run. Diet soda has zero calories, but because it contains artificial sweeteners, studies have shown that within a few years, you will be fatter than when you first started drinking diet soda.

Don't get products labeled "low fat." It's not fat that makes you fat, but rather sugar that makes you fat. Sugar gets converted straight to body fat. The body needs healthy sources of fat to stay healthy. If you're on a low-fat diet, you'll constantly be hungry because you need the correct amount of fat to feel satiated. You need healthy fat from avocados, organic extra virgin coconut oil, ghee, and nuts. Insulin is the fat-producing hormone. Insulin takes the excess sugar you ingest and puts it into your muscles. As soon as the muscles' energy stores are full, the excess sugars are converted into fat. Avoid foods that quickly convert to sugar in your body such as white bread, white flour pasta, white potatoes, muffins, waffles, pancakes, cereal, and white rice. Sugar is a drug as addictive as cocaine. White sugar should be illegal. Processed foods, especially sugar, kill more people than all drugs combined. White flour, white sugar, and high fructose corn syrup are all like cocaine—whitened, extracted, refined products taken from a natural product and made into an addictive product. Sugar and high fructose corn syrup can be found in everything. They are in pasta sauces, juice, cereal, salad dressing, and nearly every boxed, packaged food.

MSG is one of the worst ingredients found in many packaged, boxed foods, as well as in restaurant food. It's found in about 80 percent of modern food products. MSG is almost impossible to avoid. When scientists want to make a mouse fat, they give it MSG. MSG has many names; many even sound natural, and that's why sometimes it's hard to spot when you look at food labels. It can be called glutamic acid, yeast extract, hydrolyzed protein, bouillon, broth stock, malt extract, gelatin, soy protein, whey protein, and natural flavors. MSG is very dangerous because it excites the brain, causing a chemical reaction that results in addiction.

It can be hard to get enough vegetables in your diet. Vegetables are the most hated food group and yet are the most important.

Although vegetables are best consumed in their whole forms, the easiest way to get your full required serving of vegetables is to juice them along with some sweet fruits to make the juice palatable. Most people are overfed and undernourished; by juicing vegetables with fruits, they get a highly concentrated source of nutrients that are easy to digest and taste good. Many of the food labels in grocery stores are deceptive; that's why you want to buy and eat whole foods, not processed, packaged, boxed foods.

If you're upset, don't eat. That's because you're not fully aware of what you're putting in your body. People overeat when they are stressed, upset, angry, and frustrated.

THE WESTON PRICE DIET

Dr. Weston Price and his wife traveled around the world in search of the secret to health. He investigated some of the most remote areas of the planet.

He observed excellent health in many native cultures who ate specific foods. He found that their health rapidly declined once they began consuming unhealthy foods such as sugar, alcohol, processed grains, pasteurized dairy, and packaged foods. Incomplete development of the face and body, crooked teeth, and disease became common. The comprehensive research of Price as documented in his masterpiece book, Nutrition and Physical Degeneration, is unfortunately largely ignored in a country where saturated fat and cholesterol from animal sources are condemned. Through his extensive research, Dr. Price discovered that non-industrialized people do not gain weight on their traditional diets.

All traditional cultures consume some sort of animal protein and fat from fish and other seafood; water and land fowl; land animals; eggs; milk and milk products; reptiles; and insects. Primitive and traditional diets have a high food-enzyme content from raw foods such as raw dairy products; raw meat and fish; raw honey; fruits; and naturally preserved, lacto-fermented

foods.

Total fat content of traditional diets varies from 30 percent to 80 percent. Traditional diets contain nearly equal amounts of omega-6 and omega-3 essential fatty acids.

The diets of healthy primitive and non-industrialized peoples contain no refined or denatured foods such as refined sugar or corn syrup; white flour; canned foods; pasteurized, homogenized, skim, or low-fat milk; breakfast cereal; packaged foods; commercially prepared fruit juice; soft drinks; soy milk; tofu; refined or hydrogenated vegetable oils; protein powders; artificial vitamins; or toxic additives and colorings.

Dr. Price does not recommend low-fat diets, diets that restrict fat, vegetarian diets, or vegan diets. Dr. Price makes the following dietary guidelines.

Do not practice veganism; animal products provide vital nutrients not found in plant foods.

Eat only organic meat and eggs. Avoid factory-farmed meats and eggs. Avoid highly processed luncheon meats and sausages containing MSG and other additives.

Avoid rancid and improperly prepared seeds, nuts, and grains found in granolas, quick-rise bread, and extruded breakfast cereals, as they block mineral absorption and cause intestinal distress.

Avoid canned, sprayed, waxed, bioengineered, or irradiated fruits and vegetables.

Avoid artificial food additives, especially MSG, hydrolyzed vegetable protein, and aspartame, which are neurotoxins.

Most soups, sauce mixes, and commercial condiments contain MSG, even if they're not labeled as such.

Seeds, grains, and nuts should be soaked, sprouted, fermented or naturally leavened to neutralize naturally occurring antinutrients, such as phytic acid, enzyme inhibitors, and tannins.

Eat organic poultry, beef, lamb, game, organ meats, and eggs as well as wild-caught fish and seafood.

Eat whole, organic milk products from pasture-fed animals, preferably raw and/or fermented, such as whole yogurt, cultured butter, whole cheeses, and fresh and sour cream.

Use only healthy fats and oils, including butter and other animal fats, and organic extra virgin coconut oil.

Eat fresh fruits and vegetables, preferably organic, in salad sand soups, or lightly steamed.

Prepare homemade meat stocks from the bones of chicken, beef, lamb, or fish and use liberally in soups and sauces.

Use unrefined Celtic sea salt and a variety of herbs and spices for food interest and appetite stimulation.

Make your own salad dressing using raw apple cider vinegar and expeller-expressed flax oil.

Use natural sweeteners such as raw honey, maple syrup, and stevia powder.

Consume only unpasteurized wine or beer in strict moderation with meals.

Cook only in stainless steel, cast iron, glass, or good-quality enamel.

The body needs a rich supply of the fat-soluble vitamins and fat-soluble activators found in animal fats.

Many of the vitamins and minerals found in vegetables cannot be absorbed without fat, and protein cannot be assimilated without fat.

The body will rob its own stores of fat-soluble vitamins to digest protein if a sufficient amount of fat is not consumed with it, leading to nutritional deficiency.

Dr. Price recommends a diet consisting mainly of freshly ground, soaked, and fermented whole grains; grass-fed bone marrow; rare-cooked, organic, grass-fed meat; organic, grass-fed organ meats; raw eggs; wild, uncookedfish; fish eggs; seafood; nuts; seaweed; grass-fed yellow butter; grass-fed cream; tomatoes; raw/unpasteurized organic milk from grass-fed cows; and green vegetable juices made from such veggies as parsley, cilantro, zucchini, and cucumber.

To provide the body with fat-soluble vitamins he suggests making a daily smoothie with two raw eggs, one cup raw milk or kefir with two to four ounces raw cream along with some stevia for sweetness. In addition, half a teaspoon of fermented cod liver oil is taken with a quarter teaspoon "highvitamin butter oil" two to three times daily with meals.

THE MEDITERRANEAN DIET

The Mediterranean diet is one of the best ways of eating for maintaining a healthy weight and preventing disease. It has been shown to prevent age related weight gain.

A study found that the Mediterranean diet was much more effective in weight reduction than a low-fat diet. Weight reduction among participants after two years was six to nine pounds for the low-fat group and nine to thirteen pounds for the Mediterranean-diet group.

Healthy fats, which are staples of the Mediterranean diet, keep you feeling fuller longer than do diets that restrict or forbid fat altogether.

Monounsaturated fats are found in nuts and avocados. Polyunsaturatednomega-3 fatty acids are found in fatty fish (salmon, mackerel, and halibut).

According to Dr. Demosthenes Panagiotakos and Christina-Maria Kastorini, MSc, PhD, the Mediterranean diet is not only the best way to eat to lose weight, but also the best way to prevent disease. The diet is associated with lower risk for cardiovascular disease, type 2 diabetes, obesity, and some types of cancer. A 10-year study found that following a Mediterranean diet was associated with a decrease in early death rates by over 50 percent. Many people want to lower their cholesterol with diet alone. The Mediterranean diet has been shown to be a very effective method of lowering cholesterol levels and reducing heart disease risk. It's also a good alternative to drug therapy.

In combination with the Mediterranean diet, fish oil, and soluble fibers— such as psyllium, oat bran, guar gum, and pectin—have been shown to reduce cholesterol levels in multiple studies.

The lipid-lowering benefits of fish have been well known since epidemiologists noticed that the Greenland Inuit have a low coronary mortality. They eat a high-fat, high cholesterol diet, but one rich in fish, especially those containing the omega-3 fatty acids EPA and docosahexaenoic acid (DHA). It is suggested that eating two or three fish per week will prevent coronary disease. Herring, mackerel, sardines, salmon, and anchovies are especially rich in omega-3 fatty acids.

An even larger reduction in heart disease death was found among people who took fish oil capsules (900 mg omega-3 per day) instead of eating fish.

Fish oil is especially effective at lowering elevated very low-density lipoprotein (VLDL) and chylomicron levels. Fish oil has antithrombotic, antiarrhythmic, and anti-inflammatory properties in addition to lipid-lowering effects.

THE GLYCEMIC INDEX

The GI was developed by Dr. David J. Jenkins at the University of Toronto during research to discover which foods were best for people with diabetes. The GI is a numerical system of measuring how rapidly a particular food turns into sugar and how much of a rise in circulating blood sugar it triggers. With foods numbered from 1 to 100, the closer a number is to 100, the higher the GI and the more it affects blood sugar levels. The lower the GI number, the less the food affects blood sugar levels.

Foods with a GI of 55 or less are considered low, while values of 56 to 69 are medium. Those 70 or higher are high GI values. Pure glucose serves as a reference point and is given a GI of 100. High-glycemic foods are between 70 and 100 on the index and include white bread or bagels; white sugar; russet potatoes; melons; pineapple; corn and rice pasta; macaroni and cheese; corn flakes; instant oatmeal; whole wheat bread; bran flakes; puffed rice;pretzels; rice cakes; popcorn; and soda crackers.

Foods with a high GI make a person's blood sugar levels rise rapidly, which can increase the person's chance of getting diabetes. They also make managing type 2 diabetes a challenge. Foods with a low GI release glucose more slowly and steadily into the bloodstream and therefore have the lowest insulin response.

If blood sugar rises too quickly, the pancreas secretes a greater amount of insulin. Insulin helps bring sugar out of the bloodstream, primarily by converting the excess sugar to stored fat. High blood sugar leads to greater insulin release and more storage of fat. It is important to eat low GI foods to prevent weight gain and type 2 diabetes.

Research provides compelling evidence that high GI foods increase the risk of obesity. In one study, rats were split into high- and low-GI groups over 18 weeks. Rats fed the high-GI diet were 71 percent fatter and had eight percent less lean body mass than did the low GI group.

Overweight or obese people consuming low GI and low GL foods lost weight and had decreases in body mass, total fat mass, BMI, total cholesterol, and LDL cholesterol as compared to those consuming a low-calorie, low-fat diet. Study participants lost more weight even though they could eat as much as they desired. Researchers concluded that lowering the GL of the diet appears to be an effective method of promoting weight loss and improving lipid profiles.

Minimizing the consumption of high GI foods is truly one of the easiest ways to reduce your weight. Scientific evidence has shown that individuals who followed a low-GI diet over many years had a lower risk of developing type 2 diabetes, coronary heart disease, and age-related macular degeneration.

Try to avoid foods high on the GI. If your favorite food has a high GI, combine it with a low GI food to reduce the GL of the meal. Fat, protein or fiber tend to lower the GI value of the food, as they all slow the entry of sugar from a particular food into the bloodstream.

The complete list of the GIs and GLs for more than 1,000 foods can be found in the article "International tables of GI and glycemic load values" in the Diabetes Care Journal.

The GL takes into account not only how quickly a certain food is converted into sugar in the body, but also how much sugar a particular food contains. The GL multiplies the GI of a certain food by the carbohydrate content of the actual serving. A GL of 20 or more is high, a GL of 11 to 19 is medium, and a GL of 10 or less is low.

It is best to know the GI and the GL of a particular food to decide if you want to eat it. For example, the sugar in carrots and watermelon is readily absorbed into the bloodstream; therefore, they are both ranked high on the GI. People might decide to avoid carrots and watermelons because they assume that because they are high on the GI they will cause weight gain.

However, although the sugar in carrots and watermelons is absorbed into the bloodstream quickly, they don't have much sugar, so they have a low GL.

This explains why even though they are high on the GI, you will not gain weight eating small portions of them.

THE SATIETY INDEX

Researchers from the University of Sydney performed an interesting study in which they compared the satiating effects of various foods. The results of the study clearly indicated that certain foods are much better than others for satisfying hunger. The researchers concluded that the satiety index is useful for the treatment and prevention of overweight and obesity.

The satiety index measures different foods' ability to satisfy hunger. The most satisfying foods they tested were plain boiled potatoes, brown pasta, oatmeal, fish, and meat. People who consumed these foods were less likely to feel hungry immediately afterward. Foods that did the worst job of satisfying hunger were croissants, donuts, candy, and peanuts.

The satiety index is a valuable tool for those wanting to lose weight. "A diet which simply recommends cereal for breakfast overlooks the fact that muesli is only half as satisfying as porridge," says Susanna Holt, PhD. "Many health-conscious dieters will eat a meal based on several pieces of fruit and some rice cakes and then wonder why they feel ravenous a few hours later. These kinds of extremely low-fat, high-carb meals do not keep hunger at bay because they are not based on slowly digested carbs and probably don't contain enough protein. A dieter would be better off eating a wholesome salad sandwich on wholegrain bread with some lean protein like tuna or beef and an apple. This kind of meal can keep hunger at bay for a very long time." You can find the satiety index in the article "A satiety index of common foods" in the September 1995 European Journal of Clinical Nutrition.

YOU ARE WHAT YOU EAT

The common saying, "you are what you eat" is evident among all those with a "good diet" and a "bad diet." Nutrition researchers and health experts have consistently shown the dramatic difference a good diet has on a person's physical appearance, energy levels, health, and weight.

Physician and nutritionist Robert McCarrison discovered that ancient Indian races such as the Sikhs and certain Himalayan tribes had good physical development, health, hardiness, and endurance thanks to their good diet. Their diet consisted of coarsely ground whole wheat, unpasteurized milk, unpasteurized milk products, tubers, roots, green leafy vegetables, fruit, and, occasionally, meat.

McCarrison conducted an experiment on rats entitled "A Good Diet and a Bad One: An Experimental Contrast." This study reveals the health effects of the typical American diet (white bread, margarine, sugar, food preservatives).

Some rats were fed a "good diet" designed to resemble that eaten by the Sikhs and consisting of whole wheat flour, uncooked vegetables, fresh fruit,sprouted legumes, butter, fresh whole milk, and, occasionally, fresh meat. Other rats were fed a "bad diet" designed to resemble that eaten by many

Western people and consisting of white bread made from American white flour; vegetables cooked in water to which pinches of sodium bicarbonate and common salt were added; a butter substitute; processed, tinned meat; packaged jam; sugar; and common food preservatives. McCarrison showed that the rats fed a "good" diet for six months were physically efficient, healthy, strong, and active, while the rats fed the "bad" diet for six months were physically inefficient, weak, low in energy, and sick.

In his book, Nutrition and Physical Degeneration, Dr. Price documents his travels to various isolated parts of the earth where the inhabitants had no contact with civilization. While there, he studied their health and physical development. In every isolated region he visited, Price found tribes in which or villages where virtually every individual displayed physical perfection and an almost complete absence of disease—even those living in physical environments that were extremely harsh. He presented photographs in his book of primitive tribes who had a high degree of physical perfection, as well as beautiful, straight, white teeth with no decay (as compared to the teeth of "civilized" people whose diets of sugar, refined grains, canned foods, pasteurized milk and devitalized fats and oils caused facial deformities, tooth decay, and disease). The diets of the healthy "primitives" Price studied consisted of unpasteurized milk, butter, cream, cheese, dense rye bread, bone broth soups, seafood, fish, oats, fish liver, fish roe, seal oil and blubber, wild game meat, organ meat, glands, marrow, whole grains, tubers, vegetables, and fruits.

HEALTHY SUBSTITUTES

You can easily sabotage your weight loss efforts if you frequently binge on extremely high-calorie foods and high-calorie-dense foods (four to nine calories per gram), including baked and regular potato chips, croissants, cookies, French fries, pretzels, cake, and many other high-sugar foods.

If you have intense and frequent cravings that you can't control, you need to address hidden factors. Chromium deficiency is common in North America and may cause intense cravings for sugar. Candida overgrowth and parasitic infection can also cause intense hunger and constant cravings for certain foods; they are hidden factors in weight gain and an inability to lose weight no matter what you do. About 3.5 billion people suffer from parasite infections of one type or another. If you get cravings for certain high-calorie-dense junk or snack foods, replace them with healthier substitutes that are similar in taste and texture and lower in calorie density. Carob is a good replacement for chocolate. It has a similar texture and flavor but, unlike chocolate, is lower in calories, higher in calcium, and higher in fiber, and has no dairy, caffeine, or theobromine. Carob is naturally sweet-tasting, so many carob bar brands do not add sugar. Carob is also a great substitute for chocolate if you have allergies or sensitivities to chocolate. You can find carob bars at health food stores or online. For cookies, cupcakes, donuts, muffins, pancakes, waffles, brownies, cakes, pies, and all other desserts and baked goods, you can substitute a few ingredients to make these desserts healthier and lower in calorie density. The two main ingredients to eliminate are white flour and white sugar, as both have high glycemic values, causing blood sugar control problems and weight gain.

Replace wheat flour with coconut flour, quinoa flour, oat flour, spelt flour, kamut flour, rye flour, barley flour, or buckwheat flour. Coconut flour is a popular choice. It is high in fiber, low on the GI, and gluten-free.

Oat flour is another popular choice. It tastes a lot like white flour but is much healthier. It's lower on the GI and is a rich source of soluble fiber.

Replace white sugar with low GI, natural sweeteners such as pure stevia, coconut palm sugar, sugarcane juice, maple syrup, Manuka honey, and blackstrap molasses. Not everyone reacts to these sugars the same way, even if they are low in the GI, so it's best to buy a glucose meter and test your blood sugar before and after eating one of these sweeteners to see which works best for you. Calorie density is the amount of energy or calories in a particular weight of food. Generally, it is the number of calories in a gram. Foods with a lower calorie density provide fewer calories per gram than do foods with a higher calorie density. The lower the calorie density of the food, the more you can eat of it. For example, two ounces of chocolate contains 240 calories. To eat the same amount of calories in lettuce, you would have to eat 3.2 pounds of lettuce.

Diets consisting of foods low in energy density were shown to result in weight loss. You don't want to make calorie counting a religion, but try to keep within your calorie re🞔uirement range by eating mainly foods that are very low in calories per gram. You can easily look up your daily calorie intake re🞔uirements online by searching for "Estimated Energy Re🞔uirement," or use the Harris Benedict formula to estimate your daily caloric needs with respect to your average activity level.

Most overweight people have a sedentary lifestyle that includes only light physical activity associated with typical day-to-day living. The more active you are, the more calorie-dense foods you can consume. Sedentary women between the ages of 19 and 30 need no more than 2,000 calories per day. Sedentary women between the ages of 31 and 50 need no more than 1,800 calories per day. Sedentary women older than 51 need no more than 1,600 calories per day.

Sedentary men between the ages of 19 and 30 need no more than 2,400 calories per day. Sedentary men between the ages of 31 and 50 need no more than 2,200 calories per day. Sedentary men older than 51 need no more than 2,000 calories per day. Calorie density is measured by the gram, so a food's calorie density tells you how many calories are in one gram of that food. To calculate calorie density from food labels (calories per gram):

1. Get the calorie count.

2. Get the weight of the serving in grams.

3. Divide the calorie count by the weight.

The emphasis should be on the types of food that can be eaten in satisfying portions instead of on reducing the portion sizes. If you select foods that are low in energy density, you will be able to eat your usual amount of food. This will help eliminate the sense of deprivation that can accompany calorie restriction.

Conclusion

In conclusion, Thermogenic (fat-burning) pills help promote fat loss and can be useful in eliminating stubborn fat from the body. Some scientifically proven effective thermogenic include bitter orange, caffeine, capsaicin, garlic, ginger, and raspberry ketone. The fat-burning digestive enzyme lipase taken three times per day between meals along with Chinese bitter may help mobilize fat stores. There is strong scientific evidence to support the theory that dietary fiber intake prevents obesity. People who consume dietary fiber eat less and lose weight. You can also take a nonaddictive fiber supplement such as apple pectin and oat bran available in pill or powder form. The powdered forms can be added to smoothies or to recipes for baked goods such as cookies, muffins, and pancakes. Various studies have found that Hoodia gordonii is an effective appetite suppressant. Guarana is also effective in suppressing the appetite due to its caffeine content.

High cholesterol can be treated naturally with red rice extract. Gymnema Silvestre in tea form has been found helpful for those with diabetes and obesity. A daily dose of 200 milligrams of gymnema sylvestre is optimal for weight management. The phytochemicals found in various foods help prevent disease and obesity. Resveratrol (found in red wine) was shown to prevent weight gain despite a high-fat diet. Curcumin is a phytochemical found in turmeric (Curcuma longa). It promotes weight loss and prevents obesity-related diseases such as diabetes and heart disease. To prevent nutritional deficiencies and maintain your overall health, include daily supplements in your diet. Such supplements include a whole food supplement, nano-ionic full spectrum minerals, spirulina, chlorella, a free-form amino acid supplement, EFAs (wild salmon oil, cod-liver oil, or krill oil), and colonizing probiotics.

Part 2

Introduction

When looking to lose weight, the two most common areas people look at is their diet, and their fitness. Hitting the gym is a good place to start but understandably, the idea of spending hours at the gym can be deterring to some people. We all have 24 hours a day with our own responsibilities, obligations, and priorities. Our jobs, our families, our children, and our friends all clamor for attention and our time, and some of us choose to take on additional responsibilities like volunteering or getting involved in local communities.

It is no wonder that amidst all the hustle and bustle of our lives, the gym is also one of the first things we put off or drop from our schedules altogether.

After all, exercise is 50% of the equation. Our diet is the other 50% and it controls the calories we eat and if we consume less energy than we expand we lose weight. It sounds simple right? We can cut 300 kcal of energy by running three miles or we can stop ourselves from eating a bar of chocolate that we would normally eat. Between the two, not eating the chocolate bar sounds like an easier choice to make.

However, if you want not only to maximize your weight loss but to be healthy, then exercise is what you need. The secret is simple: be as efficient as possible with both your exercise and your diet.

In the first part of this book, we will look at the exercise portion of the equation. In addition to cardiovascular exercises like running, walking, and cycling you should perform some strength training exercises will help you burn more calories by raising your resting metabolic rate.

The secret to weight loss with exercise is to adopt an effective exercise routine that complements your diet. When your exercise routine and your diet work together, you don't have to spend hours at the gym a few times a week to shed a few pounds and get yourself into shape. As you can tell from the title of this book, you just need to work out while eating One Meal a Day (OMAD).

The OMAD diet would cover the second part of the book. With your diet, it should be easy to follow and satisfy you. Most dieters fail due to what is known as yo-yo dieting where people end up putting on the weight they have lost after achieving their goals. This is common because the diet that they have put themselves on is not something that they can sustain in the long run.

The One Meal a Day (OMAD) Diet is a weight loss method based on intermittent fasting, meal frequency, and meal timing. It is a way to lose fat and keep it off while eating whatever you want.

This is not a fad diet, nor is it a temporary weight loss solution. A short term diet is unhealthy and will increase your weight when you stop the diet, indeed many dieters have experienced a yo-yo effect on their weight. They do not lose enough weight to be satisfied and end up giving up their diet.

Before we go any further, I would like to make it clear that this book is not a substitute for professional medical advice. Your health is of the utmost importance and you must consult a doctor before changing your diet, especially if you have a history of medical or dietary problems. Also, when exercising, having a trainer will help to minimize the risk of injury.

Diet or Exercise - Which Comes First?

When starting out on your weight loss journey, a common question that I hear is "which comes first, should I start with diet or exercise?"

To answer this question the Stanford University School of Medicine conducted a study with 200 participants who were initially inactive in 2013. What they did was separate the participants into four groups:

1. The first group was counseled to adjust their diet and begin exercising immediately.

2. The second group was counseled to adjust their diet immediately, then work on adding an exercise routine.
3. The third group was counseled to begin an exercise routine immediately, then work on adjusting their diet.
4. The last group was a control group and did not make any changes.

The participants in this study were advised to follow the US National Fitness and Nutrition Requirements. These requirements are 150 minutes of weekly exercise, and five to nine servings of fruit and vegetables daily. In addition, saturated fats should be limited to a maximum of 10%.

What they found was very interesting:

- The participants who started dieting and exercise at the same time expectedly had the best results and were best able to stick to the recommended diet and exercise.
- Those that started exercising first before starting on their diet also managed to stick to the recommended diet and exercise but not as well as the first group.

- However, the participants who started the diet before exercising only managed to meet the dietary goals, and failed to meet the exercise goals.

When starting dietary changes, people get engrossed with the diet and are less able to motivate themselves to exercise. On the flip side, starting with exercise allows people to see a visible change in their bodies. This motivates them further to stick with their dietary and fitness changes.

Focusing on a diet change first actually interferes with establishing an exercise routine. So ideally you should begin with both at the same time or less ideally if you don't have the time or energy to make both changes, start with exercise.

Chapter 1: understanding fitness and weight loss

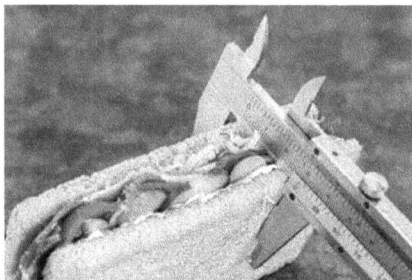

When you are starting out on your diet and exercise routine, you will naturally have many questions about what to expect. This chapter is dedicated to prepare you for the exercise portion of your new routine.

Weight Loss vs. Fat Loss

While dieting and working out, most people do not realize that there are many differences between losing weight, and losing fat.

When we lose weight, the weight that we lose can come from either essential or non-essential sources. For example, losing weight due to losing blood may not be a good thing, but losing weight from going to the bathroom may be normal. Weight loss can also come from perspiration, dehydration, diet, and exercise.

To ensure that the weight we lose is permanent and healthy, we need to lose fat. Fat is the adipose tissue that our bodies store for when food is unavailable and it needs energy to carry out our bodily processes. We need energy to live, and when there is no food our bodies turn to fat.

When we lose fat, it is typically through exercise and diet. However, fat loss and weight loss do not always happen together as we will see in the next section. This may not always be a bad thing.

Fat Loss Through Diet

When you have a highly nutritious diet with lots of protein, fat, fresh fruits, vegetables, complex carbohydrates, and nuts you will start to lose fat. These foods are low in sugar and any carbohydrates you consume are complex carbs. This will prevent spikes in your insulin levels, and when coupled with fasting (like on the OMAD diet), you will end up burning fat.

The 20 hour fasting window will put your body into ketosis, which is where your body consumes ketones produced from the fat stores in your liver instead of relying on blood glucose as a source of energy.

Once your body reaches a healthy body fat percentage it begins to use the nutrition it receives to power your body and stops storing fat like it previously did. The healthy body fat percentage is between 10% to 25% in men and 20% to 30% in women,

Fat Loss Through Exercise

Everything we do requires a surprising amount of energy, even simple tasks like walking, or carrying groceries. What more when we push our bodies with exercise?

When we work out we engage our body's energy expenditure processes, and this includes the use of our stored adipose (fat) tissues. This makes exercise or sports very effective fat loss methods because they work on two levels; by burning fat and creating tears in our muscles, which encourages it to grow.

When your muscles are damaged during exercise, this is a natural process which forces your body to use calories from food and stored fat to fuel the repair process which is how your muscles grow and how we become stronger. When doing so, your body continues to use up adipose tissue well after your work out.

Muscle is also more metabolically active than fat meaning that it burns more calories when we are at rest as compared to fat. It is estimated that muscle tissue will burn about 10 calories per pound each day, as compared to fat that burns up to three calories per pound.

Fat vs. Muscle Weight

When we start out on dieting and exercise, a common objective is to lose weight. What they often overlook is that gaining muscle will offset any fat loss at least at the beginning. Our bodies are great at adapting to changes in our diet. When we change our calorie intake we will see more weight loss in the first few weeks, but as our bodies adapt to the diet the weight loss will naturally slow down.

Also, as we exercise, we may end up putting on some of the weight that we have shed. That is because muscle tissue is denser than fat. As you begin to lose fat and put on muscle you will see that your clothing may drop a size but your weight will not change much.

However, having more muscle and less fat is beneficial to your overall health despite not losing weight. When you have less fat in your body, you lower your risk for obesity related diseases such as diabetes, hypertension, and heart diseases.

Training Frequency

When you are trying to lose fat and gain muscle it is best to have a schedule. That way your fitness becomes a priority and you will set aside time for working out.

There are many ways that people schedule their training from splitting each day by muscle groups, focusing on one muscle group a day, to splitting their workout into upper/lower body sessions, or just committing to working out three times a week. The idea here is that you must let your muscles recover from a workout before stressing it again.

Mentally has the additional benefit of making your work outs more relaxing as you do not always have to do high intensity, heart pumping, muscle straining exercises when you are feeling sore.

Rest Days and Muscle Recovery

When it comes to muscle building, it is actually your rest days that grow your muscles, not your time at the gym.

When you are exercising, your recovery is just as important as your work outs. Some trainers would argue that it is even more important as without rest your body will not recover from the stress of exercise and your muscles will not grow.

Regardless of whether you're lifting weights, running, or doing bodyweight exercises, you damage your muscle fibers and create tears in the muscles. This is normal as your muscles break down to perform physical activity.

When at rest, your muscles start to repair themselves and strengthen. This leads to larger muscles and correspondingly an increase in strength. However, muscle soreness was found to peak 48 hours after exercise therefore leading some trainers to recommend at least 72 hours of rest between training sessions but this could vary depending on your physiology, age, and diet.

Chapter 2: the science of fasting and working out

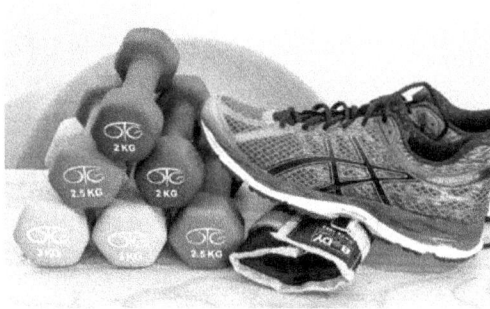

There are a lot of beliefs regarding exercising in a fasted state. There is "common wisdom" that exercising in a fasted state will cause you to lose more muscle than fat, or that eating before exercise can spike your blood sugar which would affect your performance. There are arguments both for and against exercising on an empty stomach.

So should you or should you not exercise in a fasted state?

The short answer is that working out while hungry will help boost your fat-burning potential during exercise.

Benefits of Exercising in a Fasted State

The University of Bath die a study on meal timing and physical activity in 2017, and they have found that exercising on an empty stomach improves the long term effects of exercise on our lipid, insulin, and blood sugar.

Exercise is more effective in a fasted state for two reasons.

Firstly, fasting can trigger a dramatic rise in human growth hormone (HGH), this is also known as "the fitness hormone." HGH is also secreted when we are asleep and is believed to help with anti-aging as the amount our bodies produce decreases as we age.

More importantly, HGH can also increase our muscle growth and improve exercise performance. Fasting helps you to burn body fat which increases HGH production, and it lowers insulin levels which research has shown to disrupt HGH production. After fasting for three days HGH levels can increase by up to 300%, and after a week it can increase by up to 1,250%.

Secondly, exercise coupled with the lack of food triggers our bodies sympathetic nervous system. This forces our bodies to break down the fat and glycogen that it stores, meaning we are more effective at burning fat while fasted.

When exercising in a fasted state, our bodies burn off the stored sugar and then starts to work on the fat we have stored, converting it into ketones for fuel.

There are many studies that have shown that exercising in a fasted state increases fat loss by up to 20 percent. This is because when we are not fasted, insulin is increased in our body, and higher insulin levels are linked with a slow-down of fat burning metabolism by the same amount of approximately 20 percent.

This basically means that exercising on an empty stomach makes our bodies more efficient at using fat rather than sugar as fuel giving us a better result for our effort. This is the reason that so many soldiers and marines exercise before their breakfast.

What Happens When You Fast and Exercise?

As we discussed in an earlier chapter, the Standford University School of Medicine has shown that diet and exercise have a synergistic relationship; they both help your weight loss. Diet restricts your caloric intake and increases your intake of valuable nutrients, and exercise helps to burn calories as well as build lean muscle mass. Building muscle will help to burn more calories while at rest.

On the OMAD diet, when we are in a fasted state our bodies start to use our stored fat and glycogen reserves as its main energy source to provide energy for our daily activities.

But what about when you exercise while you are in a fasted state?

A 2009 study showed that carbohydrate restriction through intermittent fasting, when coupled with exercise, can increase the endurance among trained athletes.

Exercising with low glycogen in our bodies also increases the mitochondrial biogenesis, which is the process wherein new mitochondria are formed within the cells. Mitochondria provide more energy to sustain individual cells during the workout and are known as the powerhouse of the cell.

Lastly, when working in a fasted state, the preservation mechanism of the body that protects active muscles are activated. This prevents active muscles from wasting away, which is known as muscle atrophy. Therefore, we are effectively burning our fat and glycogen stores instead of muscles contrary to popular belief.

Remember those exercise routines burn energy that supports weight loss and training under a fasted state provides some unique benefits in terms of fat loss.

Does It Affect Men and Women Differently?

Men and women have different physiologies. Therefore it is important to consider this when deciding on your workout routines during your fasting periods.

The effects of fasting among men and women are almost the same with regard to glucose and insulin response. However, Monica Klempel a researcher at the University of Illinois found that due to the menstrual cycles of women longer periods of fasting resulted in significant metabolic responses.

This includes increased production of cortisol and a disrupted circadian clock, both of which are signs of stress. In addition, there was found to be a huge reduction of LDL (good cholesterol) levels among women who maintained an intermittent fasting diet for a sustained period of time.

Dr Bajaj, the Director and Head of Medicine at the Motilal Nehru College in India has also linked prolonged fasting to early onset menopause, stress, and reproductive health issues.

But this does not mean that the OMAD diet is dangerous to women. It is important to take note that the dangerous effects of fasting among women were observed on longer and sustained fasting periods. Therefore it is important that the fasting window should be less than 24 hours, and women should discontinue fasting if pregnant, stressed, or unable to adapt to the new lifestyle.

It is important to take note that while men do not have a problem losing weight and burning off fat, it might take longer for women to see the same amount of fat being burned from their bodies. Women should attempt to approach the OMAD diet differently; their focus should be on the quality of the food that they eat, exercising regularly, and getting more sleep.

While men and women will have different experiences, they can both find effectiveness in working out on the OMAD diet.

Chapter 3: how to create your workout plan

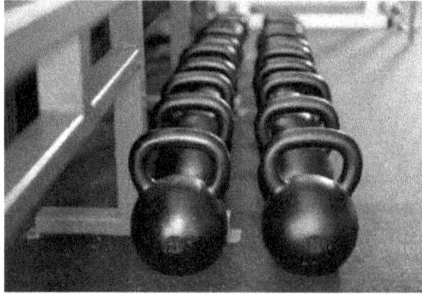

Just diet alone is insufficient for a healthy lifestyle or permanent weight or fat loss. It is important that we incorporate exercise into our routine to help our bodies shed off the excess pounds as well as to build muscle.

The challenge, however, with exercising while on the OMAD diet is that people worry that they would not have enough energy to perform their daily activities, let alone exercise. Conditioning is essential when on the OMAD diet. If you have already been exercising regularly, you would have noticed that your body burns off fat and raises your metabolism up.

When creating your workout plan may be a straightforward matter. But if you are on the OMAD diet and are frequently in a fasted state, there are additional things you would need to take into consideration. If not done properly, you may end up injuring yourself or doing harm to your body. Working out with an empty stomach should be done correctly so that you don't lose your muscle mass.

This chapter will cover the things that you need to know in order to create a good plan and exercise safely on the OMAD diet.

Start with Assessing Yourself

When you are starting out, whether it is with the OMAD diet, exercise, or both, you should start with assessing your situation. Comparing yourself to others may not be realistic, and if you are just starting out it can be downright discouraging, so then how should you assess your fitness?

One way is to see a doctor for a full assessment. This is a great option if you have leg or knee problems and intend to do high impact exercises like running, or if you have back injuries or other injuries that may affect your exercise and fitness.

Another way is to do a standardized assessment like running a mile and timing yourself or doing the CrossFit "Baseline" workout of the day (WOD). These standardized assessments can be used to benchmark yourself at regular intervals and track your progress as you improve in your fitness.

Understanding how healthy and fit you are will help you to set your expectations and goals, and help to ensure that your workout plan is suitable and realistic for you. It is also a way for you to measure your improvements over time.

The other thing you should look at is your availability. How much time can you commit? How much time do you want to commit? Remember that we all have our priorities, so you would have to set yours.

Even if it's just an hour or thirty minutes, if you fully dedicate yourself to your workout, it is better than nothing. If you plan it right, you can accomplish a lot in the time you have allocated.

Timing Your High and Low Intensity Exercises

This is the key to structuring your workouts while following the OMAD diet.

Schedule your low intensity cardio exercises during fasting periods

A low intensity cardio exercise is different for everyone as it depends on their fitness levels. Generally, you should be able to have a conversation without running out of breath while doing this exercise.

Walking, cycling, or doing simple bodyweight exercises as well as exercises that isolate and train one muscle group. These will help you to burn more fat with simple movements while minimizing the risk of you feeling dizzy.

Schedule your high intensity workouts after your meal

High intensity workouts are the ones that leave you sweaty and panting. As the name implies, they are fast paced and gets your heart pumping. To maximize fat loss, high intensity workouts should be scheduled after meals. After you have eaten, your body has glycogen that can be used as fuel.

It is recommended that you do 2 to 3 high intensity workouts during the week.

Deciding Your Workout Schedule

When you are trying to create your working routine and set a schedule, there are many things that you need to consider such as your age, biology, diet, goals, and your time available. In addition, when on the OMAD diet you will also need to consider your meal window.

If you are just starting out on the OMAD diet and working out it is crucial to determine your current situation. How much time you can dedicate for exercise and especially consider when those timings are in relation to your meal window timing.

Generally, on the OMAD diet, your fast should last 18 to 20 hours, which would take you through the night.

Most people on OMAD have their meal window in the afternoon or early evening which would give them some time to schedule a workout session before their meal. Depending on your preference, if you break your fast in the morning or early afternoon you will need to adjust your routine accordingly.

Waiting for the eating window to open may be difficult enough for some people, and having to wait for it after working out only makes it much tougher. Remember that your body needs to refuel after an intense work out.

Instead, I would suggest you consider scheduling your workout two hours or two and a half hours before your meal. Try to keep an hour between the end of your workout and the start of your meal as this is when experts believe is the post-exercise anabolic window.

The theory is that consuming nutrients an hour after exercise is supposed to be more effective at rebuilding muscle tissue and restoring energy.

Maximizing Your Workout

When looking to create your workout schedule and maximize the benefit with a limited amount of time, there are several things that you need to take into consideration.

Warm up exercises

Before starting your workout exercises you should warm up by doing static and dynamic stretching exercises. The purpose of doing these warm up exercises is to get your blood flowing and slowly raise your heart rate and breathing rate, which would help you to avoid injuries later.

Static stretching involves holding a position for 30 seconds or more to stretch the muscle while a dynamic warm up involves stretching through a range of motion.

Some examples of dynamic stretching are squats, jumping jacks, and lunges.

Select one exercise for each big muscle groups:

There are 5 major muscle groups which are the chest, abdominals, legs, arms, and back. (covered in Chapter

4), and you need to ensure that your workout plan has one exercise for each muscle group.

Perform 3 to 5 sets for each exercise

To get the most out of your workout and ensure it is effective you should perform 3 to 5 sets for each exercise with at least 10 reps per set. If you are unable to reach this number, you should slowly work your way up to 10 reps.

Diversify your workouts

You can select a different exercise for each muscle group to switch it up and keep it diversified. This keeps your workouts more interesting.

Do alternating sets or circuits

An alternating set is when you select two exercises that work the same muscle group, and you do those with a short rest between each set.

A circuit is a set of exercises that you perform one after the other, usually with a rest in between. Each exercise would work a different muscle group.

Always keep your workout short

Exercising for a longer period does not make your training more effective and may be counterproductive. The ideal exercise length should be an hour at most, which is enough for 25 minutes of cardio, and 25 minutes of muscle building exercise. Remember that you should also dedicate 5 minutes before and after to warm up and cool down your muscles to avoid injuries.

Stretch after working out

Stretching after exercise is very important as it helps improve your flexibility as well as your range of motion. It also reduces the risk of injury, particularly on the connective tissues of your muscles.

Moreover, it is also a great way to relieve the physical stress of exercising, as it can reduce lactic acid formation. This is what causes soreness of the muscles that you will be familiar with a few hours after exercise.

Chapter 4: preventing injuries during your work out

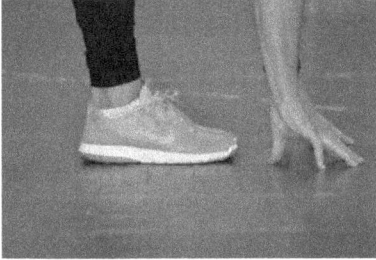

Regardless of whether you're a beginner or a pro, every person that exercises is concerned about injuries. A minor sprain may be inconvenient and affect your quality of life for a few days but anything more serious and you may lose all motivation to exercise for a long, long time.

It is therefore your responsibility to ensure that you take precautions as much as possible to prevent injuries from happening and keeping you away from your weight loss and fitness goals.

Preventing Muscle Cramps

Everyone will experience a muscle cramp. It is the sudden tightening of your muscles and it stops you in your tracks. It usually happens on your calves, but it can also happen on your lower back, abdomen, and other places where you have muscles.

Though they are generally harmless it will put a stop to your work out for at least the next few minutes. Not to mention they are also painful and uncomfortable. But what causes muscle cramps in the first place?

A muscle cramp is commonly caused by one of three things: the overuse of a muscle, strain in the muscles, or dehydration.

Less commonly, it could be due to a medical condition or a lack of minerals in your diet such as potassium, calcium, or magnesium.

To prevent a muscle cramp, you should warm up your muscles. If you are just starting exercise, you may need to take a longer period to warm up but it will be worth it if it keeps your joints flexible.

Also, you should keep your body well hydrated. If you are working out under the sun, or doing high intensity exercise cramping is more likely to occur as you are at a higher risk of dehydration.

Hydration has additional benefits which we will cover in the next section.

If you do get a muscle cramp during your exercise, understand that this is normal and will most likely go away in just a few minutes. However, you may be feeling sore a bit longer. Sit down, take a breath, and take this opportunity to hydrate yourself. You should also gently stretch the muscle, slowly at first to help loosen up the muscles. You can also gently massage the affected muscle.

The Importance of Hydration

Staying hydrated is important at all times, but it is especially important when fasting as well as before and after exercise. Since our bodies are up to 65 percent water, and our brains are 75 percent water, failing to stay hydrated could damage our bodies.

Your body will not function properly without adequate water, as it is needed to carry out its everyday processes. In fact, your body needs pure water more than it needs daily food, as you can go without food for much longer than you can go without water. We depend on water for our survival.

In one hour of exercise the body can lose more than a quarter of its water. Dehydration leads to muscle fatigue and loss of coordination. Without an adequate supply of water the body will lack energy and muscles may cramp. So, drink before, during and after a workout.

Lean muscle tissue contains more than 75 percent water, so when the body is short on H2O, muscles are more easily fatigued. Staying hydrated helps prevent the decline in performance, strength, power, aerobic and anaerobic capacity during exercise. So, when your muscles feel too tired to finish a workout, grab a drink of water before getting back to it.

The Importance of Warming Up

Before starting on your exercise routine, it is highly advised for you to warm up by doing some stretching exercises. This is also an excellent time for you to adjust your mindset, clear your thoughts, and get yourself emotionally pumped to work out.

Additionally, warming up provides you with several benefits such as:

It improves your flexibility and range of motion
As we stretch our muscles during warm up, our muscles and tendons will lengthen which will help to extend the range of your movement. This allows your joints to move more freely making your arms and legs more flexible.

It improves muscle performance
As your range of movement increases, you will find that exercise becomes easier. You are able to sustain longer work outs without feeling exhausted and you will find that your performance increases.

It helps to prevent injuries

When your muscles and tendons are well flexed and in warmed up properly, they will be able to take on more stress. You can exercise harder and for a longer period with less likelihood of injury.

It reduces muscle tension

If you perform regular warm up exercises, it is less likely for your muscles to constrict. This will definitely relieve you of any muscle pain or problems, and prevent muscle cramps. You will also experience less soreness after exercise.

Chapter 5: training the major muscle groups

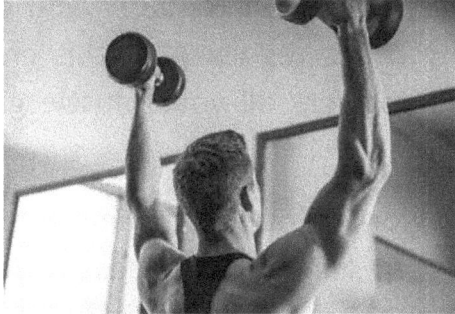

The human body has over 600 muscles which make up about 40% of your body weight. These muscles are what contracts and flexes, and are used for any sort of movement whether we are lifting bags of groceries, running for the bus, or typing on a keyboard.

However, deciding which muscle groups to train together can be confusing as a simple search on the internet would tell you. There are different trainers with many different opinions. Some believe that they should be grouped by activity such as the chest and triceps, which are used with bench pressing and overhead pressing. Others believe that they should be separated so it isolates each muscle group for maximum effectiveness.

So, how are you supposed to put all of this into an effective training routine?

All you want is a program that helps you add muscle to all the right places without requiring you to be at the gym for a few hours regularly. In this chapter I will show you how to work all your muscle groups in an hour.

When you are working out and trying to build muscle, knowing the right kind of exercises in every muscle group allows you to focus on each muscle group one at a time. This allows you to minimize injuries, prevent muscle imbalances, and build your muscles faster.

The major muscle groups are:

1. Chest
2. Back
3. Arms & Shoulders
4. Legs & Glutes
5. Abdominals (Abs)

In the next section, we will look at each of these groups and discuss the muscles as well as some exercises you can do to build the muscles in each group. With each section, there are some exercises that are bodyweight exercises meaning that you can do them without the use of gym equipment.

If you are unsure of how to perform these exercises, please consult with a personal trainer to avoid any injury or harm to yourself.

Muscle Group 1

The first major muscle group is the chest, and the main muscle group of the chest is the pectorals, also known as the "pecs" major. The chest is divided into two parts, pectoralis major, and pectoralis minor.

The pectorals or pecs are the large chest muscles. They are full of thick muscle fibers and add size to the upper body. While it does improve your physique, these muscles are used throughout the day. The main function of this muscle group is to provide support when you hold objects in front of your body and they are activated when you reach across your body.

Putting on a seat belt, combing your hair, or reaching into your back pocket are simple everyday activities that use your pectoral muscles.

To train your chest, you can do the following exercises:

- Push ups
- Bench Presses

- Chest Flies

Muscle Group 2

The second major muscle group is the back, and it is the most complex major muscular structure in the human body. It is a combination of 5 muscles that starts from above the glutes (buttocks) and goes until the neck and shoulders.

These muscles work together and complement each other to enable us to stand, reach out our arms, and pull things towards us.

The 5 muscles of the back are:

Latissimus Dorsi

The Latissimus Dorsi is also known as the "lats" or "wings" and is one of the first muscles that come to mind when discussing back muscles. A pronounced Lattisimus Dorsi has a pronounced "V" shape because of the protruding muscles under the arms and behind the ribs.

The lats enable your body to pull and compliment the arms. When you reach up and grab something off a shelf or when swimming, your lats are one of the main muscles used.

To train your lats you can do:

- Pull Ups
- Dead Lifts
- Barbell Rows

Rhomboid

The rhomboids are located in the upper back, underneath the trapezius. They not visible from outside and originate from the spinal cord and merge into the scapular bone. While these muscles cannot be seen, they strengthen the scapulae when you bring your shoulders together.

To train your Rhomboid muscles you can do:

- Pull Ups
- Barbell Rows

Trapezius

The Trapezius is also known commonly known as "traps", that are located between shoulders and the neck. The traps are a complex set of muscles and consists of upper, middle, and lower traps which extends to the lower back.

The traps control the shoulder blades (scapulae) and come into play when shrugging or moving your neck, and they provide support when you lift item above your head.

To train your Traps you can do:

- Shrugs
- Deadlifts
- Barbell Rows

Teres Major

This muscle lies underneath the lat, and it is a small but important muscle of the back. It is sometimes called the "little lat", as it works in conjunction with the lats, but also with the rotator cuff muscles.

While the teres major is usually worked in conjunction with the lats, if you want to train your teres major you can do:

- Dumbbell Pullovers

Alternatively, you can train this muscle whenever you do:

- Deadlifts
- Shoulder Presses
- Barbell Rows

Erector Spinae

The erector spinae or spinal erectors is a set of muscles that line your spinal column from your lower back to the upper back.

These muscles allow you to straighten and rotate the back and are key to maintaining a good posture. They are also important when bending your body forward, and sideways. When well developed, good erector spinae muscles will give a boost to your total strength.

To train your erector spinae muscles you can do:

- Deadlifts
- Squats

Muscle Group 3

The third major muscle group is the arms, and they are used when you use your arms or hands. They are used for four major types of movement which are: flexion, extension, abduction, adduction.

Biceps

The biceps are at the front of your upper arm and they control the motion of the shoulder, elbow, and forearm. The biceps are one of the most popular muscle group for bodybuilders, powerlifters, and especially to guys new to the gym.

The biceps are essential in lifting, especially when bending or curling the arm towards your body.

To train your biceps you can do:

- Barbell Curls
- Reverse Grip Curls
- Pull Ups

Triceps

The triceps are muscles in the back of the upper arm, behind the biceps. These muscles help to stabilize the shoulder joint and are used when the elbow joint to be straightened. Common, everyday activities that use your triceps are pushing, pulling, and using a pen.

To train your triceps you can do:

- Bench Presses
- Tricep Extensions
- Dips

Deltoids

The deltoids, or delts, are the shoulder muscles located above the biceps and have a triangular shape. They consist of 3 parts: anterior deltoid, medial deltoid, and posterior deltoid.

The deltoids are used when we flex our shoulders and help to provide support when we carry things such as groceries. When our arms are extended the deltoids help to keep our grocery bags away from our knees and thighs.

To train your deltoids you can do:

- Overhead Presses

- Shoulder Presses

Muscle Group 4

The fourth muscle group is comprised of your leg and glutes (also known more commonly as your buttocks). These muscles are one of the main workhorses of your body and you use them all the time whenever you are standing, walking, or otherwise moving around. Your leg and glutes help to hold your body up and keep your body balanced.

Gluteals

The glutes are the largest muscles in your body and form the muscles of your buttocks. These muscles help with movements of the hips and thighs, and they are key muscles that you use to move your legs especially backwards and sideways. The glutes also help you maintain balance in walking or running.

To train your glutes you can do:

- Squats
- Side Skates
- Hip Thrusts

While there are gym machines and weights to train your glutes, bodyweight training exercises have been shown to be more effective as weight machines may isolate only a single layer of your glute muscles.

Hamstrings

The hamstrings are the huge muscle group behind your thighs. These muscles help to flex your knee joints and extend your thighs behind your body. Whenever you are walking, running, or jumping, your hamstrings are being used to move your body forward by flexing. Note that the hamstrings are stretched when you are in a sitting position, so prolong periods of sitting may affect your hamstrings.

To train your hamstrings you can do:

- Romanian Deadlifts
- Squats

Quadriceps

The quadriceps (also known as "quads") are the four muscles at the front of your thighs and consists of four separate muscles originating from the femur bone and attach to your kneecaps. These muscles help in extending the knee and are used for walking, running, and jumping. The quadriceps is the second largest major muscular structure in the human body after the back.

To train your quads you can do:

- Squats
- Rope Skipping
- Lunges

Gastrocnemius

The gastrocnemius is a fancy name for your calf muscles, which are at the back of your lower legs. These muscles are used to move the heel and your feet and are used mainly when walking, running, jumping, and climbing up stairs.

To train your calves you can do:

- Calf Raises
- Ankle Circles

- Balance Boards

Muscle Group 5

The fifth of the muscle groups are the abdominals or the "abs". These muscles are also known as the core and they hold the upper and lower body together. They are a popular muscle group to train as it gives you a flatter stomach or the desired 6 pack of abs.

The abs work together with the back to support and move your torso when you twist to look behind you, or when you bend over to touch your toes. They are also used to keep your organs in place, assist with your breathing and maintain a good posture.

To train your abs you can do:

- Planks
- Crunches
- Sit Ups

Putting It All Together

So now that we have covered the muscle groups and the types of exercises that train each muscle group, let us put together an exercise routine.

When creating your workout plan, try to find balanced workouts. You should ideally have one exercise for each muscle group, and if you would like to focus on a specific muscle group you can spend a few minutes to do an extra set of targeted exercises for that muscle.

Remember that you should do 3 to 5 sets of 10 repetitions for each exercise.

5 Minutes - Warm Up
Start with 5 minutes of warm up exercises to stretch and loosen your muscles. Make sure to stretch each of your major muscle groups.

25 Minutes - Cardio
Choose one of the following cardio activities:

- Running
- Cycling
- Skipping Rope

5 Minutes - Chest

Choose one of the following chest exercises:

- Push ups
- Bench Presses
- Chest Flies

5 Minutes - Back

Choose one of the following back exercises:

- Pull Ups
- Shrugs
- Deadlifts
- Dumbbell Pullovers
- Shoulder Presses
- Barbell Rows

5 Minutes - Arms

Choose one of the following arm exercises:

- Barbell Curls
- Reverse Grip Curls
- Pull Ups
- Bench Presses
- Tricep Extensions
- Dips
- Overhead Presses
- Shoulder Presses

5 Minutes - Legs and Glutes

Choose one of the following leg and glute exercises:

- Squats
- Side Skates
- Hip Thrusts
- Romanian Deadlifts
- Rope Skipping
- Lunges
- Calf Raises
- Ankle Circles
- Balance Boards

5 Minutes - Abs

Choose one of the following abs exercises:

- Planks
- Crunches
- Sit Ups

5 Minutes - Cool Down

End with 5 minutes of cool down activity to release the tension from your muscles. Similar to warming up, be sure to stretch and relax every muscle group.

Remember that you do not have to spend hours to do this, ideally, you should be done in an hour.

Chapter 6: proper execution of exercises

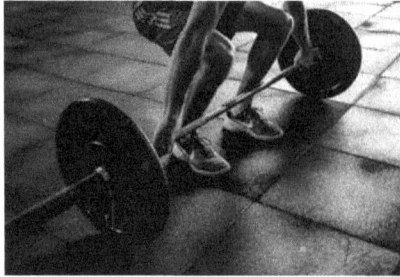

Now that you have your work out plan, you are probably wondering how to do some of the exercises, especially if you are new to the gym. The easiest way is to work with a personal trainer or to watch an exercise video on YouTube. Some of these like running and cycling are pretty straightforward, but for the other exercises that you may not know, I will try to explain here in this chapter.

You may need to use weights or some other equipment for some exercises, which I will mention where necessary. Also, I will let you know if there is anything you need to watch out for as well doing these exercises.

There are also gym machines that you can use to emulate the use of weights. These can be a great substitute for the dumbbell or barbell versions.

1. Push ups

Technique:

Start with your hands shoulder width apart on the floor and your legs together. Your body should be a straight line supported with only your arms and your toes on the ground.

Lower your body until your face is nearly touching the ground, then raise your body up using your arms.

2. Bench Presses

Equipment:
Gym Bench

Barbell

Technique:

Lie with your back on the gym bench and grip the barbell with your hands. Your feet should be flat on the ground, or if you prefer you could put them flat on the bench with your knees up.

Lower the barbell with weights to your chest until it touches your sternum.

Raise the bar to its original position.

Caution:

If you are new to this exercise you should use a spotter to help you ensure the exercise is done correctly. There is a danger of you losing control of the bar and having it fall onto your body if your muscles are not able to cope with the weights.

3. Chest Flies

Equipment:

2 Dumbbells

Gym Bench

Technique:

Lie down on the gym bench with a dumbbell in each hand.

Extend your arms directly above your chest.

Lower the dumbbells to the sides in a controlled manner until your arms are extended at the level of your body.

Raise the dumbbells in a semi circular motion until they are above your chest.

Equipment:

A pull up bar

Technique:

Grip the pull up bar and hang freely.

Pull yourself up until your chin is above the pull up bar.

Lower yourself back to the starting position.

Caution:

This exercise requires a good amount of upper body strength and is not for beginners.   Be careful when you mount/dismount the bar as they can be a few feet in the air.

5. Shrugs

Equipment:

Barbell

Technique:

Stand with your feet shoulder width apart and hold the barbell with both hands with your   palms facing towards you.

Raise your shoulders up.

Return your shoulders to the starting position.

6. Deadlifts

Equipment:

Barbell

Technique:

Stand with your feet hip width apart and bend at the hip to grip the bar.

Lower your hip and flex your knees while looking forward.

Lift the bar until it is at the level of your hips. You should be pulling your shoulders back   as the bar rises above the knee.

Lower the bar to the starting position.

Caution:

Lifting too heavy a weight can cause you to drop the weights.

When doing deadlifts, the lower back is at risk of being injured. Keep your back straight and rigid throughout the lifts.

If you are unsure of how to perform a deadlift, get a fitness coach to work with you and do not attempt this on your own..

7. Romanian Deadlifts

Equipment:
Barbell

Technique:

Stand with your feet hip width apart and hold the bar at hip level with your palms face down. Your knees should be slightly bent.

Lower the bar by moving your hips backwards as far as you can. Keep the bar close to your body at all times and face forward.

Slowly return to a standing position by moving your hips forward.

Caution:

Lifting too heavy a weight can cause you to drop the weights.

When doing deadlifts, the lower back is at risk of being injured. Keep your back straight and rigid throughout the lifts.

If you are unsure of how to perform a deadlift, get a fitness coach to work with you and do not attempt this on your own..

8. Dumbbell Pullovers

Equipment:

A dumbbell

Gym Bench

Technique:

Lie on the gym bench with your shoulders on the surface. Your feet should be planted   firmly on the floor.

Hold the dumbbell with both hands over your chest and extend your arms outwards   above your body. Your hands should both be holding one of the weighted ends of the   dumbbell.

Keep your arms straight and lower the weight in an arc until the dumbbell is behind your   head.

Raise the dumbbell back above your chest.

Caution:

Always secure the weights to the dumbbell.

If you are new to this exercise you should use a spotter to help you ensure the exercise is done correctly. There is a danger of you losing control of the bar and having it fall onto your body if your muscles are not able to cope with the weights.

9. Shoulder Presses

Equipment:
2 Dumbbells

Technique:

Sit on a bench or chair with back support with your feet firmly planted on the floor.

Raise your dumbbells to ear level with your elbows slightly bent. The dumbbells should   be parallel to the floor. Your head should be resting against the back support.

Raise your arms up and touch the dumbbells lightly over your head.

Lower the dumbbells back to ear level.

10. Barbell Rows

Equipment:
Barbell

Technique:

Stand with your feet under the bar and bend over to grab the bar with both hands.

Lift your chest and straighten your back while lifting the weights to shin or ankle height.

Pull the bar against your chest.

Lower the bar back to shin or ankle height.

Caution:

Keep your blower back neutral to avoid back injuries. Do not round or lift with your back.

Put the bar on the ground between reps if it is too heavy. This will help to prevent injury   as well.

11.Barbell Curls

Equipment:
Barbell

Technique:

Stand with your back straight and legs about shoulder width apart and hold the barbell in   both hands with your elbows close to your body. Your palms should be facing outwards.

Keep your upper arms and shoulders in place while using your biceps to lift the weights.   Only your forearms should be moving.

Lower the barbell slowly.

12.Reverse Grip Curls

Equipment:
Barbell

Technique:

This is similar to the barbell curl (above) but you grip with your palms facing your body.

Stand with your back straight and legs about shoulder width apart and hold the barbell in both hands with your elbows close to your body. Your palms should be facing inwards.

Keep your upper arms and shoulders in place while using your biceps to lift the weights. Only your forearms should be moving.

Lower the barbell slowly.

13. Tricep Extensions

Equipment:
Dumbell

Technique:

Stand with your feet shoulder width apart and hold a dumbbell with both hands.

Slowly lift the dumbbell over your head until your arms are fully extended and your palms are facing upwards.

Keep your elbows close to your head and lower the dumbbell behind your head. Your forearms should touch your biceps when complete.

Lift the dumbbell over your head with your arms fully extended and your palms face upwards.

14. Dips

Equipment:
A benche

Technique:

Position yourself between 2 benches perpendicular to your body.

Put your hands on the bench behind you and hold the edge of that bench.

Lower your body slowly by bending your elbows and keep your elbows as close as   possible.

Lift your body back up again.

Equipment:

Barbell

Technique:

Grip the barbell with a wide grip and position the barbell behind your neck and above   your shoulders. The bar should not be resting on your body and should only be   supported by your hands.

Keep your elbows under the bar and extend your arms with the barbell overhead.

Lower the barbell behind your neck and just above your shoulders again.

16.Squats

Equipment:
Barbell (optional)

Technique:

Stand with your feet slightly wider than your hips. Point your toes outward.

If you choose to use a barbell, you should hold it behind your head, above your   shoulders. If you are not using a barbell, you should keep your arms straight in front of   your body for balance.

Push your hips backwards as you bend your knees while keeping your back straight and   looking forward. Keep squatting until your hips are lower than your knees.

Reverse the motion and push your hips in while straightening your knees.

17.Side Skates

Technique:

Stand on a mat in a half squat position.

Jump sideways to the left side. When you go to the left, land on your left leg and put your right leg behind your left ankle without touching the floor.

Jump to the right side and land on your right leg. Put your left leg behind your right ankle without touching the floor.

18.Hip Thrusts

Equipment:

Gym bench

Technique:

Begin by sitting on the ground with a bench behind. Put your arms on the bench and lean back so your shoulder blades are near the top of the bench.

Drive your hips upwards using the feet. You may have to tiptoe to get the full motion. You should finish with your body bent only at the knees, and parallel to the ground.

Relax and lower your body.

19.Lunges

Technique:

Stand upright with your feet apart and your knees unlocked.

Take a step forward with one foot and lower the knee of your other leg. Your body should be upright and your knee should be off the ground. The front leg should have its knee bent at a 90 degree angle.

Push back up with your front foot and step back, bringing your knee of the other leg back beside the other.

Repeat with the other leg.

20.Calf Raises

Technique:

Stand with the ball of your feet on the edge of a step. Your heels should be unsupported.

Raise your heel above the step so that you're on tip toes. You can hold this position for a while if you like.

Lower your heels back to below the step.

21.Ankle Circles

Technique:

Steady your body using a wall, chair, or some other object and lift one leg in the air.

Perform a clockwise motion with your toes, like you are drawing a circle with it.

Repeat with the other leg.

22.Planks

Technique:

Lie on the floor and lift your body up. Support your weight using your toes and your forearms. Your elbows should be bent and below your shoulders.

Keep your body straight at all times and hold this position.

23.Crunches

Technique:

Lie on your back with your knees bent and your feet firmly on the floor. Put your hands beside your ears or behind your head. Your elbows should be facing outwards.

Curl up and bring your knees up and your elbows forward at the same time. They do not need to touch.

Relax and lie back with your knees bent and your feet on the floor.

Technique:

Lie on your back with your feet secure and your knees bent. Put your hands beside your   ears or behind your head. Your elbows should be facing outwards.

Raise your shoulders and torso towards your knee, ensuring that your elbows touch the   knees.

Relax and go back to lying on your back.

Chapter 7: the omad diet

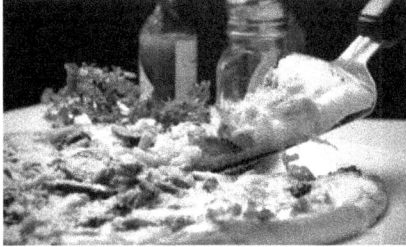

The One Meal a Day (OMAD) Diet is a weight loss method based on intermittent fasting. The main principles of this are regulating your meal frequency, and meal timing. This is a proven way that many people have used to lose body fat and keep it off.

Note that this is not a fad diet, nor is it a temporary weight loss solution.

Most diets are short term and result in a yo-yo effect where people actually lose weight but then they are unable to keep themselves off a pizza or chocolate bar. They end up caving in to their cravings, or they are unsatisfied with the weight loss that they have achieved. Either way, they end up giving up on their diet and some even gain more weight than they have lost while on a diet.

The issue is that these diets do not address the root cause of weight loss, which is to manage the circadian rhythm. This is done by timing exercise, meals and sleep which is managed when we stick to the rule of 4 "Ones" of the OMAD diet which will be covered in this chapter.

The reason the OMAD diet works is because it is a lifestyle and one that works for the long term because it is based in science. If you can follow the plan you will improve your health, energy, and well being. You do not have to count calories, worry about what you can or cannot eat, and mostly you do not have to feel guilty for cheat days.

Starting the OMAD Diet

While eating one meal a day may sound simple at first, there is a recommended approach to this diet. Like any other diet, the beginning of the switch in eating habits will require conscious effort to maintain, and you will need to build on this consistently in order to achieve long term success. When you are consistent in your daily eating habits, the diet starts to take effect and help you achieve the weight loss that you have set out for yourself.

The basis of the OMAD diet is the rule of 4 "Ones".

In essence, this means you should have:

1. One Hour
2. One Meal
3. One Plate
4. One Beverage

This rule helps you to maintain the discipline and have a structure to your diet. Many people have found this method to work best for weight loss, as well as maintaining a long term healthy lifestyle. So how do you follow the Rule of 4 Ones?

One Hour

When starting the one meal a day diet, you need to choose a four hour window to eat. This can be any four hours you want, but make sure it will best fit into your schedule as it would be best to stay consistent with the eating window.

Once you have chosen your four hour window, you should allow yourself one hour for your meal so you have sufficient time to enjoy your food which can include a beverage of your choice. When the hour is up, there should be no more calorie intake until the next eating window.

When choosing your eating window, it might take some time to figure out how to choose the best one to fit your situation, but maintaining a structure will make all the difference in your weight loss journey.

One Meal

Each day, you will have a 4 hour eating window but you should only give yourself 1 hour in those 4 hours to eat. In that one hour, you will have only one meal.

In the OMAD diet, there should be no small meals or cheat hours where you can eat snacks or junk food.

The only exception to this is for protein shakes taken post workout. If you do workout, these protein shakes are necessary to fuel your body with protein.

One Plate

Since you are restricted to one meal, it may be tempting to pile on whatever you want in your one hour window. When you are eating your one meal, it's important to understand what is going on your plate and ensure that there is a balance of nutrients, proteins, and carbohydrates.

It is recommended to incorporate a serving of vegetables, carbohydrates (potatoes, rice, or bread), protein and fats (from meats), and a serving of fruits. The caloric intake for most people during OMAD is around 1,500 Kcal.

An average sized plate could actually hold two servings of meals so it is important that you make an informed choice of what goes onto your plate and not overeat during your one meal.

One Beverage

During your meal, you should allow yourself to have one beverage of your choice. This can be anything you crave, from beer to a soda, or anything else you want. This serves as a perk me up to boost your mood. The OMAD diet is not about depriving yourself, it is just a structured way to approach your food and drink intake.

Taking a drink with a caloric count can also help you to get your calories required for the day, but you should keep yourself to one serving.

Apart from this, you should continue to hydrate yourself by drinking water throughout the day. You do not have to limit your intake of water. Tea and coffee can also be drunk at any time, as it may help to suppress your hunger.

What to Expect When Starting OMAD

When starting out on OMAD diets, the most common thing that people experience is hunger, as one would expect, so know that you are not alone. This is most likely an issue of body conditioning that you will have to battle the first few weeks. You may not actually be hungry, but because you have been eating several times a day, your body has been conditioned to expect food every few hours. This is something that everyone on the OMAD diet would have to push through.

While this will vary from person to person, a "fasting headache" is common for the first few weeks at least. This is triggered by a combination of low blood sugar, dehydration, and possibly lack of sleep. The trick is to stay hydrated throughout your fast as it will help to ease the headaches and hunger pangs.

The brain is 75% water and is very sensitive to dehydration, and produced histamines to ration and conserve water when faced with a shortage. It is these histamines that cause headaches as well as fatigues; they are a signal that we need to drink more water. Keep in mind that this discomfort will end once your body gets used to your new eating schedule and the lack of intermittent snacks throughout the day.

Another good way of keeping hunger at bay is to keep yourself busy with work or distracting yourself with other activities. This will help you keep your mind off food. Consciously staying away from the kitchen or the pantry will also help as you will not be constantly seeing and smelling food to whet your appetite when it is not your meal time. Out of sight, out of mind.

Once your mind has been disciplined to eat only meal a day, your body will adjust eventually.

Chapter 8: breaking your fast post work out

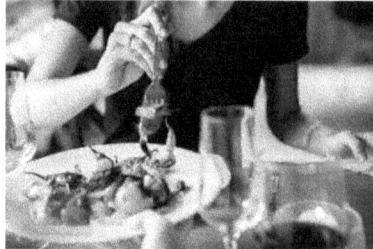

When you are on the OMAD diet, your post workout meals are very important. Since you will be exercising on an empty stomach, there is an anabolic window after your workout. This is when your muscles are receptive to nutrients, and this period lasts anywhere from 1 to 3 hours after your workout. It is therefore very important that you break your fast at most one hour after your workout so you can fuel your body and rebuild your muscles.

What to Eat when Working Out

If you're on the OMAD diet and want to build muscle bulk, a high amount of protein is necessary for muscle synthesis. When we exercise, our muscles are broken down and they need to repair themselves throughout the day. This is how they grow, and protein is necessary for this to happen.

Bodybuilders have a rule of thumb where they take 1 gram of protein per pound of their body weight. When trying to lose fat, some bodybuilders can increase that ratio to 1.5 grams per pound.

Studies have shown that the ratio of protein intake to bodyweight is roughly 0.13% to 0.18%. Meaning that you need about 0.2 - 0.3 ounces of protein for every pound you weigh although other factors such as the intensity and frequency of your workout, your age, and your gender can affect this.

Healthy fats such as nuts, seeds, avocado, cheese, and dark chocolate are also a great source of fuel for your body. Increasing your intake of healthy fats also helps to decrease cravings, which would prevent you from going hungry after exercising.

Aside from proteins, carbohydrates are another important part of our diet. It is recommended that we eat whole-grain cereals (with low-fat or skim milk), whole-wheat toast, low-fat or fat-free yogurt, whole grain pasta, brown rice, fruits, and vegetables when working out on the OMAD diet. These are more complex carbohydrates that take longer to be digested, and help to stave off hunger as well as reduce the spikes in our blood glucose.

Sugars and grains are also carbohydrates but should be avoided as much as possible along with processed food. These foods cause cravings as well as our blood sugar to spike severely which overworks our body's digestive system. After the "sugar rush" also comes a crash in blood sugar which brings about hunger and the craving for more food.

Remember that our bodies are different, and we all adjust to routines differently. When making any changes to habits, introduce them slowly and give it some time to take effect and show results otherwise it will lead to frustration.

The important thing is that we are consistent with our diet, our eating window, and our workout routine as the OMAD diet is a lifestyle.

Also, you must remember to hydrate yourself before and after your work outs. This has been mentioned several times in this book, but the effects of dehydration can be severe. Exercising while dehydrated has been linked to kidney failure, seizures, and even death.

When Should You Eat? Post or Pre Workout

When you are trying to build muscles you will need to provide your body with protein and amino acids. These are the building blocks of your muscles which you will need to repair the muscles and enable them to grow after exercise.

Post work out, it is important that you break your fast and get nutrients to your muscle cells as fast as possible. When you elevate your insulin levels it will help to drive nutrients to your cells.

In this situation, carbohydrates are especially important as they are depleted when you exercise and need to be replaced. High protein foods like red meat are also necessary as they will easily satisfy your body's requirements for nutrients as they are easily assimilated into the cells of your muscles. Lastly, you might also want to consider adding healthy fats such as avocado, cheese, or fatty fish. These healthy fats help to keep your blood sugar more stable and do not cause an insulin response in your body so including some healthy fats in your meals will help to decrease food cravings.

This would be an ideal post workout meal to break your fast.

While the post-workout meal is important, it is also essential for you to consider pre-workout meals as sometimes you will need to work out after your meal or you may feel less dizzy and fatigued if you eat something before your work out. If you choose to exercise after your meal you should still consume something like a high protein or high (healthy) snack after your exercise.

Note that this is not strictly OMAD, but remember that we all have our individual physiologies so you should do what works best for you. If you feel unwell or uncomfortable at any time during your fast, you should stop fasting and try again once you feel better.

A pre workout meal or snack will help to stimulate protein synthesis when you are exercising. This will prevent muscle breakdown when you are exercising. A study conducted in 2014 found that fasting for at least 10 hours puts the body in fat metabolism while avoiding muscle catabolism at the same time. When you eat before exercise, especially if you are planning a high intensity workout, it gives your body the energy it needs.

Planning your meal pre or post workout is crucial when on OMAD. You can opt not to have a pre workout meal but you should never skip the post workout meal, even if it's just a snack.

For most people, a 20 gram protein bar or shake before working out can help with fat burning as well as promote muscle growth. Remember that you are trying to lose fat and gain or maintain your muscles, not lose it. Other options are to eat some Greek yogurt with berries or nuts, hard boiled eggs, or a low carb granola bar.

The most important thing when deciding your approach is to listen to your body. If you feel weak or dizzy when exercising on an empty stomach, stop your exercise and eat something. Your health and well being should be your priority, and your body will adjust to your fasting and exercise routine over time.

Principles When Planning Your Post-Workout Meals

There are several things to consider when you are planning your post workout meals in order to get the most benefit out of it. Below are some guidelines I use when I am planning my meals and exercise routines.

1. Fast for at least 20 hours daily.
2. Strictly eat within the 4-hour feeding window.
3. Exercise with a high intensity workout twice week while in a fasted state.
4. Consume at least 10 grams of protein before exercising.
5. During your exercise days, consume a meal comprised of protein, vegetables, and small amounts of carbohydrates.
6. During non-exercise days, eat a meal of protein, vegetables, and fats. Consume only whole and minimally-processed foods.

While this may not suit everyone due to our personal preferences, different physiologies, and individual schedules you can use this as a starting point and adjust them to your needs.

Maybe you need to have a larger feeding window, or you may require more protein before your work out. Try it out, adjust what doesn't work, and adopt what works best for you.

Chapter 9: nutrition on omad and exercise

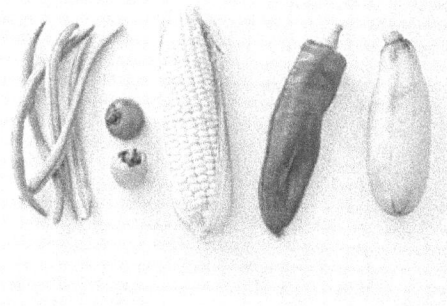

Now that we have discussed when to eat your meals, in this chapter we will be looking at what to eat during your meals. While when we eat is important on the OMAD diet, what we eat determines how we look and feel. After all, it is commonly said that "we are what we eat".

There are many studies on nutrition when exercising and they all point to the fact that the food we choose to eat is just as important as exercise if not more important than exercise. A well balanced meal is an important part of a healthy lifestyle, especially when combined with exercise.

The 3 Main Nutrients

The foods that we eat will have different effects when we exercise while in a fasted state. Our bodies will have different reactions when we have a huge amount of carbs and not enough protein or vice versa. It is therefore important to understand the types of food that you should eat to complement your workout routine and help you achieve your dieting and fitness goals.

Carbohydrates

Carbohydrates are found in almost all foods and provide 4 calories of energy per gram. Foods that contain carbs basically fall into two types:

1. Simple Carbohydrates:

These are also called sugars and are made from glucose, fructose, and galactose. Because the chains of these carbohydrate molecules are short they are easier to break down and are easily digested and absorbed into the bloodstream.

Foods such as sugar, honey, jellies, jams, as well as products made from flour like white bread and cake contain simple carbohydrates.

2. Complex Carbohydrates:

Complex carbohydrates come in two forms and are either a starch or a fibre. While they   are made up of the same sugars as simple carbs, complex carbs have an additional   sugar molecule with a longer chain. This makes complex carbs more difficult to break down and digest. This slows down the absorption into the bloodstream, which prevents   insulin levels from spiking.

Brown rice, wheat and wholemeal bread, beans, and vegetables are all examples of   complex carbohydrates as are bananas and berries.

When you are on OMAD, it is beneficial for you to choose complex carbohydrates, especially those that contain high fibre. Vegetables and whole grain are examples of high fibre complex carbohydrates. Since they take longer to break down in your body, these will keep you full for a longer time and also prevent spikes in your blood sugar.

When on exercise you should take some carbs, it is after all the preferred fuel source for your body. Carbs are what fuels your workouts, although if you overload on carbs and do not burn off the excess calories they will be stored as fat in your body. One of the reasons we are seeing more obese people is because their calorie consumption is higher than their energy output.

When choosing **carbohydrates** you should consider:

- Whole grains
- Oatmeal
- Brown rice
- Sweet potatoes
- Bananas

- Pears
- Apples
- Oranges

Protein

Protein is a key component of every single cell in our bodies. They are made up of amino acids which are essential for growth and the repair of broken down tissue - which is the result of exercise. Additionally, the amino acids found in protein cannot be produced by our own bodies. Since our bodies cannot produce its own protein, they must be supplied by our the food we eat.

When we do not have enough protein, our bodies are put in a catabolic state where it tears down our muscle tissue to meet its protein needs.

While protein is also a source of energy like carbs and fat, it has many other functions as well, and it cannot be converted into fat and stored in our bodies like carbs. For that reason, the body digests carbohydrates and fat first before protein to get energy.

That is why we need to eat protein when working out. We want to lose fat and gain muscle, and not the other way around.

When choosing protein, a lean cut of beef or pork like tenderloin or chuck can reduce the calories you gain from fat. Plat based protein, fish, or poultry are also good alternatives.

When choosing **proteins** you should consider:

- Lean beef
- Chicken
- Turkey
- Fish
- Eggs
- Low fat dairy

Fat

Fat has an undeserved reputation. There is a common belief that eating fat makes you... fat. However, fat is not always a bad thing as it has many benefits aside from just making your food taste good. Fats are a very dense source of energy, holding 9 calories per gram. That is more than double what you get from carbohydrates.

In addition, fat can contain many nutrients such as essential fatty acids such as omega-3 and omega-6 which support your nerves and respond to inflammation. Fats also contain cholesterol which is used to keep your cells healthy. Note that too much cholesterol can lead to heart disease, and if you lack this in your diet your body can manufacture the cholesterol it needs. Lastly, fats also contain vitamins. Notably, vitamins A, D, E, and K.

Fats are composed of building blocks called fatty acids, which fall into four main categories:

1. Polyunsaturated

Polyunsaturated fat are also found in animal and plant oils. These are healthy oils and can lower your LDL cholesterol (bad cholesterol) levels. These include omega-3 and omega-9 acids that is needed for brain and cell function. Note that polyunsaturated fat is not produced by our bodies.

While polyunsaturated fat is consider healthy, it should also be consumed in moderation. If reducing your blood cholesterol is a health goal, eliminating saturated fats is much more effective than increasing your consumption of polyunsaturated fats.

Polyunsaturated fat can be found in corn oil, sunflower oil, fatty fish, flax seeds, and walnuts.

2. Monounsaturated

Monounsaturated fat is found exclusively in plant foods such as olives, nuts, avacados, and vegetable oils. These are also healthy fats that can help lower your LDL cholesterol, similar to polyunsaturated fat.

A way to tell the "healthy" fats apart from "unhealthy" fats is that Saturated fats and trans fats are in a solid state when at room temperature. Monounsaturated fat and polyunsaturated fat are in a liquid state at room temperature, but will harden to a solid when chilled.

3. Saturated

Saturated fats are found in animal and dairy products as well as some plant based oils. Saturated fats when consumed can be processed by the liver to make cholesterol which is then used to produce hormones in our bodies. Consuming some fat in our diet helps to keep our body's hormone levels up at optimal levels.

Foods that have saturated fat are: whole milk, cheese, red meat, coconut oil, and vegetable shortening.

4. Trans Fats

Of all the types of fats, trans fat is the worst of the lot. Too much trans fat poses a risk for heart disease, but we need to understand the difference between naturally occurring trans fat, and the processed trans fat.

Natural trans fat can be found in some meat and dairy products such as beef and lamb. These are less of a concern if you choose low fat or lean cuts.

Processed trans fats occur when polyunsaturated fat such as vegetable oil is made into a solid like margarine through a chemical process called hydrogenation. This changes the physical properties of the fat such as the melting point, which is desirable when mixing with flour for baking. However this has a side effect on our health and can manifest as circulatory or heart disease.

Thankfully, the food industry are moving away from processed trans fats and using other sources of fat in our food. Trans fats are also frequently found in labels on food packaging.

In general, fat intake should be kept low when you are working out and trying to put on muscle. In fact, many bodybuilders practice eating "clean". That is sticking mainly to lean meats, dairy, and complex carbohydrates, with the option of adding supplements of omega-3 to get their recommended dosage of healthy fat.

Most foods are a combination of all saturated, unsaturated, and monounsaturated fat, although one is typically the dominant type which therefore dictates it's classification.

When choosing **fats** you should consider:

- Flaxseed
- Sunflower seeds
- Canola oil
- Olive oil

When choosing **fats** you should avoid or reduce:

- Processed vegetable oils
- Butter
- Lard
- Margarine

The Nutrient Ratio You Need for Weight Loss

When we are trying to lose weight through diet and exercise, we want to not only need to output more calories than we take in, we would also need to make smart choices on what to eat and what not to eat in order to achieve our goals. This will help us to reduce our fat and replace it with muscle which helps to set our bodies up for a higher resting metabolism. This means that our bodies will burn more calories while at rest when we have more muscles.

As we learned in the earlier part of this chapter, carbs are an important source of fuel for our muscles and it is also the only source of energy for our brain and red blood cells. Fat helps with brain function and cell development. Lastly, protein is used to build and repair muscle tissue. Therefore, not all foods are equal. We want to consider how much of these 3 nutrients we want to take in order to support our goals.

When you are on OMAD there are additional considerations because your feeding window is very small. You will need to make the right food choices to get the most nutritional value in your one meal and keep in mind the rule of 4 "ones". With your one plate you should be aiming for 1,500 calories- 2,000 calories for men, and between 1,200 calories - 1,500 calories for women.

Protein is necessary, and arguably the most important component of an OMAD diet. The recommended dietary allowance for protein is 0.36 grams per pound of bodyweight. That means for an average person who weighs about 165 pounds, you will need 60 grams of protein per day. However, when you are exercising you will need more. For an average person again, the protein intake should be easily doubled. Cutting down on protein means that you won't get enough amino acids which will put you in a catabolic state, causing you to ultimately lose lean muscle.

Fats in our diet are just as equally important as they regulate your hormones and your thyroid. The recommended daily allowance of fat is 15% of your daily calories but on OMAD it is recommended that you increase this to at least 20% which is about 40 grams of fat on a 2,000 calorie diet. If you are going low carb, or even keto it should be even higher. Some people have managed to maintain a diet of up to 150 grams of fat and stay healthy. Just remember to choose healthy, polyunsaturated or monounsaturated fats.

Carbohydrates are the least important of the three nutrients. While the recommended daily allowance for carbs is 50%, restricting carbs often have a positive effect on weight loss. When choosing your carbs, you should make healthier choices as far as possible.

Remember that this fruits such as apples, bananas, berries, and vegetables all have carbs but they are all healthy choices as they contain vitamins, fiber, and other nutrients. If you choose to have pasta, rice, bread, or other flour bread products a multigrain option is more beneficial for you.

If you exercise often and have an active lifestyle, then having more carbs in your diet may not be a bad thing. Still, you can do OMAD with minimal carbs or without carbs at all, but it is not optimal as you will be missing out on a lot of vegetables, fruits, and other plant based foods. While you can survive on a zero-carb diet it should ultimately be your personal choice.

Lastly, there is no magic ratio for everyone. The optimal ratio is largely dependent on our individual physiologies and whether there are any health problems like type 2 diabetes or problems with our metabolism. The beautiful thing, however, is that on the OMAD diet you don't really need to obsess over this. It is certainly good to keep in mind your ratio of protein to fat to carbs but most of all you should enjoy the foods you eat and make a conscious choice to eat healthily and enjoy your meals. When you have a healthy relationship with food it will definitely impact your health and weight in a positive manner.

Chapter 10: supplements while working out on omad

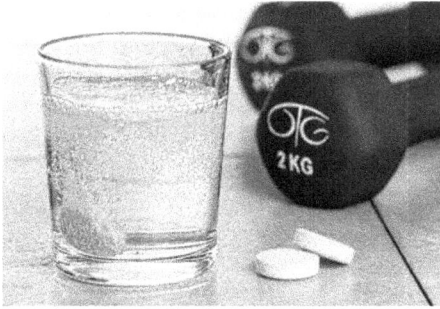

Our bodies need a certain amount of essential vitamins and minerals to function, and many people will tell you that you should supplement your meals when fasting. However, the truth is that you don't need to have a constant stream of vitamins in your body.

Most of your minerals are stored in your bones, fat, liver, and other places. When you fast, your body will break down and catabloze the dead cells and start to use up the nutrients that are stored up. However, this only occurs if you fast for long periods of over 48 hours.

Just to be clear, you do not need to take any supplements on OMAD.

Choosing to take supplements, however, is another issue. If you are on a high protein, high fat diet, then having some supplements can help you balance your meals and achieve better overall health. Some supplements can also help when you are fasting and working out. Consuming these would definitely help you maintain your fast and get the most benefit from your exercise.

With supplements, you need to consider your medical condition, metabolism, and the type of supplements you want to take. It is best to check with a pharmacist or a doctor, especially if you are on any medication when adding supplements.

BCAAs

First let's get one thing clear about Branched Chain Amino Acids (BCAA): They will break your fast.

So what are BCAAs? They are an amino acid with a different "branched" structure of carbons that allow our bodies to transport BCAAs from the liver to the bloodstream directly.

BCAAs are supplements that contain amino acids, which are the building blocks of protein. They help keep our muscles in a non-catabolic state and also help support endurance while working out as well as improve the muscle recovery.

But more than boosting the endurance and building muscles, amino acid supplements also reduce fatigue, increase fat loss, and also improve the cognitive function of the brain. Moreover, it also has anti-inflammatory properties and can remove inflammation on the joints and muscles.

There are 9 amino acids in total, but the main ones that BCAAs contain are Valine, Leucine, and Isoleucine.

BCAAs have a caloric value of 6 Cal per gram and will trigger an insulin response in our bodies because they contain proteins. Since fasting is meant to keep your insulin levels low, taking BCAAs will break your fast.

BCAAs are present in the food we eat and you can get them if you eat foods such as whey, casein protein shakes, eggs, beef, chicken, and fish.

Taking BCAAs are said to protect against muscle loss. However, they've been shown to be effective only if you exercise in a fasted state. Taking BCAAs while fasting will also give you extra energy, and if you are pushing yourself during your work out you may be able to perform better and get more fat loss or muscle gain.

Casein Protein Powder
Similar to BCAAs, casein will also break your fast.

Casein is a slow digesting dairy protein consisting of 80% milk protein. This means that it feeds your cells with amino acids over a long period of time.

A lesser known fact about casein is that it helps to synthesize protein, even when your body might be breaking down its own muscles. This happens when fasting, and it makes casein beneficial for an OMAD diet as the slower digestive process keeps the amino acids in your body longer.

In addition to the above, there are some more benefits found in research on casein:

- **Antibacterial and immune benefits:** casein may provide antibacterial and immune benefits as well as reduce high blood pressure.
- **Fat loss:** fat loss is improved by three times when on casein
- **Reduction in free radicals:** peptides in casein protein powder may have antioxidant effects.
- **Triglyceride levels:** casein reduced triglyceride levels after a meal by 22%.

Creatine

Creatine monohydrate is a performance enhancing supplement that is popular among athletes and bodybuilders. It can improve your cells' ability to produce Adenosine Triphosphate (ATP) which provides energy for your muscles. It is believed to improve strength, increase muscle growth, and help muscles recover during exercise. This is especially so during short periods of intense activity such as weight lifting.

So what happens when you take creatine when fasting?

Unlike casein and BCAAs, creatine will not break your fast as it does not contain calories. In fact, it is popular with people who practice fasting in one form or another.

However, to get the full effects of creatine you will need to combine the effects of creatine with insulin as it will produce greater results. Creatine acts as a buffer for liquid retention and inhibits fluid absorption. That means that your muscle holds more water which will impact your muscle performance when insulin and creatine are present in your body at the same time. In a fasted state, creatine is still absorbed but it will take more time.

If you do want to take creatine, you should take it with your meals and workouts. Creatine doses of 5 grams daily are more than enough to reap the benefits and improve your physical performance and help you build muscle.

Multivitamins

Multivitamins provide the necessary elements so that your body can carry out different physiological functions. When you are on the OMAD diet, you may want to supplement your meal with a multivitamin that provides you with your daily requirements of vitamins. As you are only eating one plate of food it may not be possible to get everything on that one plate all the time.

Multivitamins are a sure way to get your daily requirements of vitamins and minerals that your body needs.

Some vitamins are easier to absorb with food, while others work fine when fasted. When you take vitamins on an OMAD diet you will need to experiment with what works best for you. If you feel dizzy or weak when you take your vitamins you may need to change your schedule.

If they upset your stomach or make you feel dizzy, you may need to moderate them. You should pay attention to how you feel and how your body reacts to the multivitamins you are taking. Over time, you should find out what works best for you.

Healthy Fats

While there are many types of fat supplements on the market, the main supplement is fish oil which contains high amounts of omega-3 fatty acids. Fish oil comes from the tissue of cold water fishes as they generally have a higher fat content.

Examples of these fish are salmon, anchovies, sardines, and tuna.

Taking a fish oil supplement helps to improve our blood pressure, blood lipids, and heart rate. Aside from the cardiovascular benefits, It also serves as an anti-inflammatory agent. These findings are from a study published by the Mayo Clinic in 2017.

When choosing a fish oil to take, you should look out for one that is purified and free of heavy metals and other harmful toxins.

L-Carnitine

L-carnitine is a naturally synthesized amino acid that is produced in our bodies when we burn fat and remove toxins in the cells. Since it is naturally produced and our bodies make enough for our needs we would almost never encounter a deficiency in this compound unless we have a medical disorder or are on some medication, usually kidney disease.

There are claims that L-carnitine can help with fatigue, improve athletic performance, and improve heart health. However, all of these currently lack sufficient evidence as the research is still in the early stages. Despite what many others may claim, this is not backed up by science at the moment.

There are very likely no side effects from taking L-carnitine, but just as likely no benefit to most people. If you wish to take this supplement, I would recommend discussing with your doctor first.

Vitamin D

This is a fat soluble vitamin that helps your body to absorb calcium and phosphorus which is important for your bone health and can prevent osteoporosis. It can be made by our bodies when our skin is exposed to sunlight which includes vitamins D1, D2, and D3. As a supplement, vitamin D is best taken after food although it can be taken on an empty stomach as well.

A study by the British Journal of Nutrition in 2008 has linked vitamin D supplementation with fat loss and proposed a link with a calcium specific appetite control for obese women.

In 2011, a group of German researchers published a paper on PubMed that links vitamin D supplementation to the testosterone levels in men. Vitamin D was found to benefit the male reproductive tract and have a positive effect on the prostate.

Iodine

Iodine is a supplement that is needed in our bodies. We usually get it from our food intake since this cannot be naturally produced, but there is very little iodine in food unless it has been added during processing. Sea kelp, or seaweed, is the best known source of iodine, but strawberries, eggs, and yogurts contain some as well. However, if you need to supplement iodine it is best that you take it in the form of capsules.

While on the OMAD diet, there is no additional reason to supplement iodine in our diets other than the fact that iodine deficiency is a common health issue worldwide.

Chapter 11: myths on nutrition, exercise, and fasting

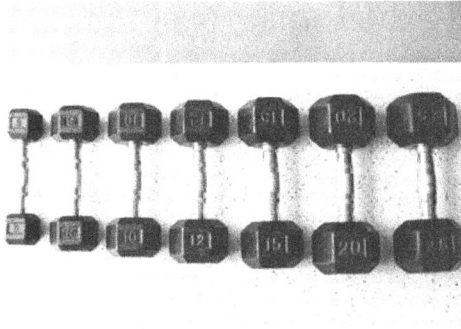

Mainstream nutrition is filled with myths and half truths usually passed down from old wives tales and folk wisdom. Even in this day and age as nutrition science advances, I am still amazed by the beliefs that some people have on nutrition. Now add fasting into the mix, and that adds a whole dimension to the myths.

However, when you are serious about getting in shape false beliefs and bad information can do harm to your body. It pays to be informed with the facts so here are some of the myths that you need to know about nutrition, fasting, and exercise.

Myth: Our body cannot absorb more than 30 grams of protein

One of the most common myths on protein is that our bodies cannot absorb more than 30 grams at a time.

It has been shown in a 1999 study published in the American Journal of Physiology that consuming protein in excess of 40 grams after exercise can stimulate muscle growth. Consuming a high amount of protein helps to stimulate muscle growth and reduce muscle loss and nowadays many athletes and bodybuilders around the world have adopted this practice.

It has also been found in other studies that if you consume more protein than your body needs, the rest will just be excreted the next time you go to the toilet. Your body will store and take up the amino acids and use it where it is needed by the body and the rest is disposed.

While you may consume more than 30 grams of protein on a meal especially on OMAD, it is not something that you should worry about.

Myth: Cutting carbs will make you skinny

A low carb diet has been a well established method for quick weight loss, but this can actually backfire. When you cut carbs from your diet your body goes into an energy deficit.

When this happens, it can have an effect on your energy, mood, appetite, and gut function in the long term. A low carb diet is one which often results in yo-yo dieting as people make up for the lack of energy during the day by overeating.

In fact, cutting carbs causes weight loss through losing water instead of fat. Carbs support the thyroid glad and can assist in providing energy when exercising. So instead of cutting carbs, it is recommended to choose complex carbs or fruit and vegetables as a healthy carb option.

Myth: Eating carbs makes you fat

Carbohydrates serve and important function such as replenishing your body's stores of glycogen. It also helps you to feel full and according to a 2002 study, carbs are also responsible for improving the quality of your sleep.

While our bodies need carbs we need to take it in the right amount and from the right sources. Healthy carbs, such as whole grains, vegetables, fruits, and other complex carbohydrates taken in moderation is a good thing.

Of course you can choose to go low carb or remove them from your diet altogether (with the support of a nutritionist or a doctor) but it is not mandatory for weight loss.

Myth: Eating fat makes you fat

Fat contains more calories per gram compared to carbs and proteins. This gives it the reputation of causing weight gain. What people fail to realize is that fats are a necessary part of our diets just like carbs and proteins. They all do their part to keep our bodies healthy and they all play a role in our physiologies.

Foods that are high in healthy fats have higher calories and they help to keep us full for a longer period. This helps to control our cravings as there is no insulin spike which means that we do not experience a sugar crash.

It is important that we eat the right fats in the right portions and take a balanced approach to nutrition.

Myth: You can eat as much as you want and whatever you want when you break your fast

The OMAD diet has the rule of 4 "ones", and one of them is restricting you to one plate of food.

This does not mean that you can stack the pizzas on your plate until it starts to fall over. The idea of having one plate is to restrict your portion while ensuring that you have a balance of proteins, fats, and carbs. An average sized plate could actually hold up to two servings of meals therefore you need to make an informed choice of what goes onto your plate.

You should not overeat just because you only have one meal as tempting as it may be.

Additionally, it is recommended to incorporate a serving of vegetables, carbohydrates (potatoes, rice, or bread), protein and fats (from meats), and a serving of fruits. You should aim for a caloric intake around 1,500 Kcal. The key to successfully losing weight on the OMAD diet is to eat normally when breaking your fast. Eating 3 meals in 1 negates the time you spent fasting.

Myth: The longer you spend working out the better

This is the myth that quantity can replace quality, and this myth has been around for a long time. It may seem obvious that the more time you spend working out, the more your muscles will grow.

However, what is more important than the length of your workout is using the right technique and the right intensity for your fitness level. If you have a clear objective with your training you can easily get your workout done in an hour.

This is supported by a paper in the American Physiological Society, published in 2007. It was found that repetitions of shorter exercise can help to metabolize more fat. Breaking a work out into smaller work outs with a rest period in between was found to be more beneficial.

The American College of Sports Medicine has also recommended that the exercise duration should be between 45 minutes to 60 minutes.

Myth: Eating OMAD causes muscle loss

There is a belief that when we fast our body will start to use our fat as fuel. While this happens with any diet, there is no evidence to suggest that it happens more with OMAD or any intermittent fasting diet as compared to other diets.

A study published in the Obesity Reviews in 2011 found that an intermittent caloric restriction caused the same amount of weight loss as a continuous caloric restriction, but with reduced loss in muscle mass.

Another study published by the American Journal of Clinical Nutrition found that eating one huge meal in the evening with the same amount of calories they were used to will actually help people lose body fat and increase muscle mass.

This means that having One Meal A Day is actually more beneficial than other diets with regards to minimizing muscle loss. In addition to that there are additional benefits to fat loss and other health markers.

Myth: Eating one meal a day is bad for your health

A study conducted by the National Institute of Aging concluded eating one meal a day rather than three, decreases your insulin resistance and helps your glucose intolerance. These are both features that are related to type 2 diabetes.

OMAD actually enhances your body's hormone function to facilitate weight loss. When you fast your body adjusts by having lower insulin levels, higher growth hormone levels and increased amounts of norepinephrine. These all help to increase the breakdown of body fat which is then converted into energy.

The American Journal of Clinical Nutrition found that fasting actually increases your metabolic rate by 3.6% to 14%, which helps you burn even more calories.

There are also many other studies that correlate fasting with a longer life spans and improved health.

Myth: Eating OMAD will make you gain weight

While a big meal may have a correspondingly huge amount of calories, you will be in a calorie deficit while fasting. Eating a big meal does not change that as your body will be burning more calories than you take in.

Additionally, research has shown that eating a big meal before you start fasting can preserve muscle mass better when compared to other diets. As long as you stick to the rule of 4 "ones" you will not put on weight by following the OMAD diet.

Myth: Fasting will slow your metabolism down

Since you are eating less often when you fast, it is a common fear that your metabolism will slow down when on OMAD. This is a common myth that has been debunked by the Journal of the Academy of Nutrition and Dietetics in 2015.

The American Journal of Clinical Nutrition have shown in studies that fasting for 48 hours will improve your metabolism by up to 14%, but longer fast will slow your metabolism. Also, fasting on alternate days for a 22 day period does not decrease your metabolic rate but may cause you to lose 4% of body fat.

Remember that the OMAD diet is not about calorie restriction and it is not about denial of your favorite foods, it is about restricting the time in which your body gets its calories.

Myth: I should eat my meal in the morning/afternoon/evening

On the OMAD diet, you can eat your meal anytime that you wish during the day.

There isn't a best or optimal time during the day when eating one meal a day so you should consume your meal whenever it is most convenient for you. Consistency is the key to getting the best results on OMAD. We recommend choosing an eating window that best fits your lifestyle and schedule.

If you are exercising, it is alright to have a snack before your work out if you need to and then break your fast 30 minutes after exercise. Alternatively, you could have your meal first then exercise an hour after that. If you do this, you may want to have some protein after to help your muscles grow.

The only suggestion would be that you leave a few hours after your meal to digest your food before going to bed as it will make you feel less uncomfortable.

Myth: Fasting for 20+ hours a day and eating one meal will give me gastrointestinal distress

We all know that our stomachs have acids to digest and break down our food, and it is a misconception that when there is no food our stomachs will devour itself.

When there is no food in our stomachs the epithelial cells will start to secret mucus and bicarbonate to protect itself and become less acidic in the process. It will adapt to having less food or no food.

Since you are eating only one meal a day, your digestive system isn't as overworked as before. If you reduce highly processed and fatty foods, digestive issues will be reduced even further. Your gut microbes get more diverse and you increase the tolerance against bad microbes which will reduce inflammation of the gut.

If you have gastrointestinal issues the OMAD diet can help because you will not constantly be trying to process food in your gut.

Eating OMAD improves your gastrointestinal health.

Myth: OMAD will negatively impact my mood and energy levels due to hunger

When we fast two things start to happen to our bodies.

Firstly, fasting increases the growth and development of brain cells and nerve tissues. Dr Mark Mattson, a Neurology Professor at John Hopkins University has found that fasting increases the growth and development of brain cells and nerve tissues. Additionally, fasting has also shown to reduce inflammation in the brain which can lead to Alzheimer's and other neurodegenerative disorders.

Secondly, our bodies learn to look for alternate sources of energy such as our fat stores. When we eat once a day our metabolism also changes and our bodies start to use fat instead of food as energy. As fat is slowly digested and sent to the liver for processing it happens steadily over a longer period of time and does not cause spikes in our blood sugar and has less effect on our metabolism.

This is in line with what other people who fast have reported in terms of increased concentration, and better memory. This also results in being more mentally stable and alert during daily tasks.

Myth: All diets restrict calories and OMAD is the same

184

The daily caloric intake for men is roughly 2,500 kcal and for women 2,000 kcal.

However on OMAD you do not have to count your calories as long as you stick to the rule of 4 "ones". The structure of the 4 "ones" ensures that you will get sufficient calories without overeating, but also allowing you the luxury of your favorite foods.

You can eat until you are feeling full, but know that you will get hungry around your regular eating times. At the start this can be tough, but a good way to gauge is to drink some water and wait for an hour or two. If you're still feeling hungry, then consider breaking your fast.

If you are tracking what you eat for building muscle, then tracking your macros is a totally different issue.

Myth: I will be constantly hungry on the OMAD diet

This is a very common question and usually the first to come up when I mention that I only eat once a day. The thing is, when you are on the OMAD diet it will become easier the longer you stick to it.

Your body is used to eating three times a day, and maybe with snacks in between, and it has learned to expect food at certain times. The hormone known as ghrelin is responsible for making us feel hunger, and has been found to peak around meal times.

When you fast you can expect ghrelin levels to continue to peak around meal times, especially during the first week. This eventually will pass as your body adapts to your new routine. There are some people who have reported that during their meal windows, they don't even feel hungry. You should give your body time to adapt accordingly as it will take you some time to get used to OMAD.

When starting a fast, drinking water will help to combat the hunger. Some nutritionists explain that the hunger may be dehydration or boredom as eating three times a day is a habit that we have been conditioned with all our lives. Drinking unsweetened coffee and tea may also help with hunger similar to drinking water.

When you are first starting out, it can be tough, but keeping a positive and disciplined mindset will help you achieve success in your diet. Everyone is different as to when your body will adapt to your new lifestyle.

It is alright if you do not follow the OMAD diet every day, you can and should break your fast if you feel unwell, dizzy, or if it is interfering with your daily lifestyle. You can always try again when you feel better.

As with any diet, it's a marathon and not a sprint. Although it is called a "diet", OMAD is actually a lifestyle change and brings with it many benefits.

Discipline is a huge factor in succeeding with the OMAD diet, and it can be difficult at times to deal with the discomfort and the hunger, especially in the initial stages. If you have to break your fast early or take more than one meal it is okay.

This is a long term thing, and it takes time for your body to adapt. There are many people who have tried OMAD and failed many times before succeeding. Some of them do OMAD only once a week or on alternate days.

To be successful, you just have to stick with it and don't give up. Once you start to see the benefits that self discipline has brought you, you will be more determined to push forward and get the success you wanted.

Conclusion

Thank you for taking the time to read this book!

By now I hope that you have taken action on your fitness or diet routine at least. Once you put the information here to use, your physique will improve along with your health and fitness. Exercise and OMAD together will have tremendous effects, but even if you adopt only one of them you should still see a result that you would be satisfied with.

The next step here is to consult with your doctor and a fitness instructor, begin planning your meals and workouts, and starting on your journey. If you can, take action today; the longer you put things off the more likely you are to continue procrastinating.

Set your goals, adjust your mindset, and take action.

If you have enjoyed this book and want to learn more, please do have a look at my other book on the OMAD diet.

Train safe, eat healthy, and enjoy your meals!